A Life of Struggles

Memoirs of
Kundan S. Khera

PublishAmerica
Baltimore

© 2003 by Kundan S. Khera.

First printing

ISBN: 1-59286-619-0
PUBLISHED BY PUBLISHAMERICA, LLLP
www.publishamerica.com
Baltimore

Printed in the United States of America

Dedicated to my wife Claire.

Acknowledgements

I extend my heartfelt gratitude to my wife, Claire Paulin, who was extremely generous with her time and help in all phases of developing this book, the seemingly endless word processing, editing, formatting, and proof reading. Her faith in me never faltered. To my brother, Surat, I give sincere thanks for his critique, photographs, and research into Punjab's revenue records, which provided valuable data for the text.

I am grateful to so many people for their help with this project: my friends whose cooperation was absolutely essential, Clyde Sanger, Douglas Fisher, and Gordon Barrow for their encouragements and useful criticisms, Rowena Beamish for editing the manuscript, Joseph Duhamel for the graphics, and PublishAmerica for making this publication a reality. The following libraries were extremely helpful in my research: St. Petersburg Public Library (Main Branch), University of South Florida Health Sciences Library, Ottawa Public Library (Main Branch), and National Research Council (CISTI) Library.

About the Cover

North Cape is located on the extreme northwestern tip of Prince Edward Island where the westerly flowing waters of the Northumberland Strait meet the eastern currents of the Gulf of St. Lawrence. At the meeting point lies a strip of land projecting deep into the ocean with its level hardly above the surface of the water. The strip, strewn with rust-colored stones, is constantly struck by the opposing waves of the Strait and the Gulf. Walking to the end of the strip when the tide is rising is an awe-inspiring experience. This rocky path with tidal waves closing in from both sides is a befitting illustration of the journey of my life.

Cover art: Joseph Duhamel, Avalon Design Unlimited.

Postscript

Kun's journey came to a sudden end on April 1st, 2003 when his ailing heart failed. CP

Contents

Introduction

Two memorable events marked the major achievements of my career. The first was my nomination by the Society of Toxicology, an organization of over 3,000 scientists worldwide, to receive its 1988 Arnold J. Lehmann Award for scientific excellence and continued contributions to the science of toxicology.[1] The second, just as surprising but far more significant, was my selection as one of the 2,000 outstanding scientists of the 20th century by the International Biographical Centre in Cambridge, England.[2]

As a child walking through the dusty streets of Punjab on my way to school, I never dreamed that I could ever reach such heights. The journey from those streets to the peak of my career has been one long, arduous struggle.

My birth was very special to my parents because I was their firstborn and more so because I was a boy. It was even more special to my maternal grandparents. They had so desperately wanted a male child of their own but had eight girls. A girl, under Indian law at the time, could not own or inherit land. So, my grandfather saw me as a potential heir to his farmland, even though he had already mortgaged most of it to nurse his opium and alcohol addictions. My widowed paternal grandmother also rejoiced. I would carry on the family name. Four of her sons remained unmarried, as they were too poor to attract anyone. My father was her only son married at the time. His military-sponsored veterinary education had turned out to be a trump card in wooing my mother's parents.

How did I who had once been wanted so much by so many go wrong? This was very much on my mind when self-awareness hit me at the age of 18. My life was dismal and disorderly. I was about to enrol in first year (grade 11) of Punjab University for the third time after wasting two years running away from a schizophrenic father who had been relentless in his verbal abuse. Plus, he wanted to control my life and had succeeded in getting me married

---

[1] Please see *Toxicology and Applied Pharmacology* (1988).

[2] International Biographical Centre, *2000 Outstanding Scientists of the 20th Century,* Second Edition 2001, Cambridge, England.

at age 15. I would soon be a father myself. Worse was the poverty: it stalked me like a shadow. I was so traumatized and confused that the thought of making my life a worthwhile experience seemed ludicrous.

I was bitter and angry with everyone, but more so with myself. I was depressed, yet I knew I had to turn my life around and find my way in the world. Fortunately, I had two assets that enabled me to initiate a process of self-healing: I was given to reflection and thought even as an adolescent, and I was a voracious reader. Reading gave me comfort and understanding. The life and teachings of Gautama Buddha became a source of moral principles and compassion; yoga inspired in me hard work and self-discipline. These values were my guiding light.

A number of events in India influenced my life. I experienced India's struggle for independence firsthand: I lived through the *Satyagrah* – the movement of passive resistance to British rule – public rallies building momentum for freedom and peaceful and not so peaceful demonstrations; I heard political leaders incite the public with exhortatory speeches, which often resulted in hunger strikes, racial riots, and death, *lathi* (baton) charges by police, and on-again, off-again Indo-British negotiations for India's independence. National newspapers, particularly those written in India's native languages, spewed out articles which often exaggerated alleged atrocities by British authorities while overstating the courageous resistance of Indian freedom fighters. Hungry for news, people concocted and circulated their own rumors, speculations, and predictions. Fact and fiction mingled indiscriminately.

I feel fortunate to have lived in the times of Mohandas Gandhi. I well recall an incident that was reported in the newspapers in September 1931, concerning Gandhi's visit to England. He had been invited to the Second Round Table Conference on India's freedom. While there, King George V invited him to Buckingham Palace where he was entertained by the King and Queen Mary. They served him Indian fruit on golden plates (Chaudhuri, 1987). Ghandi, dressed in simple Indian garb – a homespun *dhoti* (loin cloth) and hand-made sandals – was his usual humble self. His unassuming demeanor and unusual appearance caught reporters by surprise. They were further stunned when England's foremost politician, Winston Churchill, refused to meet Gandhi, referring to him as "this half-naked Fakir from India." India was deeply offended by Churchill's demeaning remarks directed at this man of peace and non-violence.

Soon after the end of World War II, when newspapers in India were filled for weeks with court proceedings on the trial of the Indian National Army (INA), I like many others felt a strong sense of identity with its personnel. The INA, aided by the Japanese, had fought the British forces in Burma in an effort to gain India's freedom from colonialism. After the INA's surrender, the trial began. All the officers and soldiers of the INA were imprisoned in the Red Fort of Delhi. The question deliberated by Indian justice was whether the INA's fight to free India from British domination was a legally acceptable act or an act of treason against the Crown. Day after day, newspapers presented arguments and counter-arguments made by the most prominent defense lawyers who, grasping the historic significance of this opportunity, rendered their services gratis. India's politicians and its future prime minister, Jawaharlal Nehru, set out on a whirlwind speaking tour of India to unite the nation firmly behind the captured INA. National emotions ran high, with crowds chanting one slogan in one voice, "Set them free!" The mounting crisis in India was moving toward the brink of a revolution, leaving the British no other choice. All INA nationals were freed.

On March 2, 1946, prior to the declaration of India's independence, Master Tara Singh, our enigmatic Akali Sikh leader, created considerable excitement in front of the Punjab Legislative Assembly by unsheathing his *kirpan* (traditional sword) before a large crowd and shouting "Death to Pakistan!" in a display of defiance (Singh, 1966). This ominous precursor of events to come would soon ambush the Indian nation and its journey to independence.

Upon independence in 1947, the resulting partition of India and Pakistan into separate and distinct Hindu and Muslim states produced a transmigration of the population on a tragic scale never before witnessed by the world – Muslims from India to Pakistan, Hindus and Sikhs from Pakistan to India. Thousands of people on both sides of the border walked or traveled by train to the safe side of the newly created Indo-Pakistan border. Hundreds of thousands of innocent people were massacred en route – Hindu and Muslim alike. Following partition, incidents occurred at lightning speed, zigzagging between frenzy, euphoria, bloodshed, and tragedy. India was consumed with action and excitement, and I was in the midst of it all.

As was the case at the time with many others my age, we were attuned to the birth of political events evolving into the independence of India from colonial rule. We belonged to politically oriented students' unions and were highly interested in the freedom of our country. Once independence was achieved and law and order established, we did not assume that an immediate economic miracle would occur. However, we did expect, perhaps naively, fair and equitable treatment from the government consistent with the tenets of democracy. We hoped that officialdom would treat its subjects with the dignity and respect to which all human beings are entitled.

Sadly, this never happened. The leaders of the bureaucracy were the very same individuals who had been the obedient servants of the colonial rulers and who had already been rewarded for their loyalty to the previous regime. They were, in fact, the calcified remnants of the colonial system and, with few exceptions, incapable of developing or adjusting to the new egalitarian form of human relations. Their presence dominated the new bureaucracy. Wily and unscrupulous subordinates abounded whose ingratiating conduct manipulated the new management by stoking their vanity and telling them whatever they wanted to hear. Thus, the end became more important than the means, adulterating ethical standards of fairness and justice. Such was my new India.

Large numbers of students sought to study abroad where devotion to study would be rewarded. Those with first-hand knowledge of conditions in India never returned. Many who did return were soon disillusioned with the prevailing culture of cronyism and nepotism. Many among them left India forever, and I was one of them. And so, I escaped the deeply ingrained malaise of Indian society that had adversely affected, not only my own career, but also my father's 31 years of service in Punjab's civil service, and thwarted any chance I had of succeeding in my homeland.

In 1964, I chose Canada as my new home, my new country, where I worked for 28 years with the Food and Drug Directorate of Health Canada. Since my retirement in 1992, I have had ample time to reflect and to record the people and events that have shaped my destiny. In writing my biography, I had to rely to a large extent on personal observations and events that had an impact on my life. I also drew on conversations with my father and other relations, especially my brother, Surat, who is now retired and resides in Ludhiana, Punjab.

Throughout my research, I strove for accuracy, corroborating events with independent sources whenever possible. Memory is fallible. The impact or individual perception of events may be subject to alteration with the passage of time. Details may be lost, but as the intensity of emotions fades, oftentimes events become clearer and may be viewed with greater objectivity.

Chapter 1: My Roots

A family that has forgotten its past is not any different than a country that has not recorded its history.

My Ancestors

My ancestors passed on to me a part of their chromosomes, their name, their village, and their land. They gave rise to a community organized territorially, a community closely knit with blood ties, almost tribal in some respects, which developed in me a strong sense of identity and belonging.

My earliest known ancestor, Bahar Singh, and all his descendants were Sikhs. A monotheistic faith, Sikhism promotes personal relations with God through prayer, meditation, and recitation of hymns consistent with the scripture in *Guru Granth Sahib,* the holy book of Sikhs. All Sikhs hold in reverence the teachings of the ten Gurus, or religious teachers, who succeeded each other from 1469 to 1708. The ninth Guru, Tegh Bahadur, was executed by the Mogul Emperor Aurangzeb, in Delhi on November 11, 1675. His execution and the religious persecution of Sikhs and Hindus left no choice other than to take up arms. His son, the tenth Guru, Gobind Rai, baptized Sikhs on April 13, 1699 to a new brotherhood, *Khalsa,* meaning "pure." He gave the hereditary name Singh (lion) to males, Kaur (lioness) to females, and five emblems to the *Khalsa: kesa* (hair), *kangha* (comb), *kacch* (knee-length short), *kirpan* (sabre), and *kara* (bracelet). Sikhs never cut their hair, always wear long shorts and a bracelet, and carry the traditional sword and a comb. They are also advised not to smoke and to refrain from drinking alcohol.

I encountered many obstacles in tracing my roots. Birth, death, and marriage records either did not exist or were lost. Funerals, cremations, and population census were often conducted without permanent records. While land tax and revenue documents were available, they were either incomplete or did not date back beyond 1700. In northern India, *Pandas* used to maintain written ancestral data. They also performed other functions, such as bearing the ashes of loved ones for dispersal in the River Ganges. Decline in this religious custom, however, contributed to the *Pandas'* demise, and it is now extremely difficult to either locate these individuals or retrieve their data.

A summary of Punjab Revenue records, dated June 16, 1893, handwritten in a mixture of Urdu and Persian and partly illegible, was a source of invaluable information. Aside from outlining the method of revenue collection and the amount of revenue in rupees, it provided me with the names of our male ancestors: Bahar Singh Khera was the first or the earliest known generation, and my father, Kesar Singh, was the ninth generation. The earliest migrants to our village seem to have been Bahar Singh and three of his four sons: Jagat Singh, Bhagat Singh, and Gurdass Singh (see chart). They came from the small village of Manoki, which is about 35 miles away. The name of the village has since been changed to Manakdeke and is still inhabited by Khera families.

The arrival of Jagat and his father can only be estimated as around 1715.[3] The village then belonged to *a kanungo* named Govardhan Lal, who had founded it earlier, possibly when Mogul emperors encouraged the reclamation and cultivation of wastelands to enhance their revenue. In all probability, Govardhan Lal was an assignee of Emperor Aurangzeb, who ruled India from 1658 to 1707.

The *kanungo*, usually a hereditary position and the designated government official, collected land revenues and maintained local land records. The village of Kot Govardhan Lal was named after Kanungo Govardhan Lal and had most probably been assigned to him by a Mogul emperor. The bulk of Punjab's cultivated land during the Mogul era was in the hands of so-called assignees, who were either contractors for the army, civil officers who assisted the government, or headmen who collected land revenues. These assignees were given land estimated to yield an income adequate to their salaries or services. They made periodic payments to the ruler in the form of cash or valuable gifts as a sign of dependence, respect, and obligation. The amount by which their revenues exceeded the tribute was their remuneration.

The system of assignment became unpopular during and after Aurangzeb's rule, which was marked by social and political turmoil. Land revenues were raised to unaffordable levels. Peasants absconded, and lands were abandoned. François Bernier, a French physician at Mogul courts,

---

[3] Calculations: 1895 (probable year of Father's birth) less 180 (9 generations x 20 years for an average generation) = 1715.

described existing conditions as "execrable tyranny." Assignees had difficulty realizing the expected remuneration due to the scarcity of peasants and because the system of assignment was in decay (Hague and Burn, 1963). Large farmers and landholders called *zamindars* replaced assignees at the end of Aurangzeb's reign. They maintained a fighting force, had authority over local areas, and provided protection which the Muslim Empire could no longer provide. Each landholder collected revenues from the peasants under his power and remitted them to any superior authority strong enough to insist on payment.

These were the existing political conditions when Jagat bought the Kot Govardhan Lal land for an undisclosed amount. He had been a co-owner and long-term lessee for an unknown period of time before the purchase. He was joined soon after by his third brother, Umar Sahai, and Amir Singh Khera (relation unknown). The village afterward became known as Kot Khera.[4]

For the purpose of revenue collection, eight family lines (*patis*) were officially recognized as equal owners of the Kot Khera land: Jagat's grandsons, Jassa, Bahar, Bhagail, and Hazara; his brother Umar Sahai; Amir, Allah Dad, and Jiwan. Allah Dad and Jiwan were Muslim blacksmiths, who had cultivated the village lands for a long time. Of these eight family lines, only the first five paid taxes to the two Sikh governments, Ramgarhia and later Ranjit Singh. The two blacksmith *patis* were not mentioned later, since their descendants sold their land to the Khera clan in the 19th century.

When Emperor Aurangzeb died in 1707, Punjab was thrown into a long period of chaos and anarchy marked by either inefficient or short reigns of a succession of puppet kings in Delhi from 1708 to 1738, followed by Nadir Shah of Persia (1739), Adina Beg (1739-1758), Marathas (1759), and Ahmed Shah Durrani (1761-1767). The first four generations of our ancestors lived through this period of lawlessness, presumably in a state of chaotic security until 1767, when Sikh rule brought some semblance of peace and order.

Subsequently, Maharajah Ranjit Singh suppressed Sikh rule in 1799 by capturing Lahore and, in 1802, Amritsar, the headquarters of Sikh rulers.

---

[4] The spelling of my village name, Kot Khaira, and of my family name, Khera, although different in records, should be the same. "Khera" is the spelling of choice of most of the families I have met. It is also written this way by the Punjab Revenue Department in its map of the Baba Bakala Tehsil (county). Khera, then, is used to denote both the village and the family name throughout the present text.

Ranjit amassed a formidable force of horsemen comprised of 50,000 each of disciplined soldiers and well-armed militia (Griffin, 1963). The militia was recruited to supplement the regular army in an emergency. Ranjit gave *jagirs* or land ownership to a militiaman for his services to the state and maintenance of his horse.

According to the *jagir* register at Nawan Shahr, the headquarters of Tehsil (county), 27 Khera families from Kot Khera were granted *jagirs* on August 6, 1808, obviously during Ranjit Singh's rule. The total number of Khera families residing in Kot Khera at that time was about 54, meaning that about half of our ancestors were in Ranjit's militia. These *jagirs* were located in different villages of the above Tehsil. Our family's *jagir* was in Mangowal, and Mehar (see chart, p. 198) was most probably the initial recipient.

It is not known whether Mehar moved to Mangowal. However, his only son, Nihal, like the descendants of other *jagir* holders from Nawan Shahr, joined Ranjit's militia and took up permanent residence either in Mangowal or in whichever village their *jagir* was located. Some of them still owned land in Kot Khera, which was good pasture land of wild grasses, or "swank." This militia would stop by Kot Khera on their way to Amritsar for annual military training and let their horses pasture for a few days.

After Ranjit's death in 1839 and the Anglo-Sikh War of 1843-1849, some of our ancestors from Nawan Shahr stayed on while others moved away[5] or returned to settle permanently in Kot Khera.

My Legacy

My great-great grandfather, Nihal Singh, died in the Sikh wars of 1848-49 while fighting against the British army. He left a teenage son, Jawala Singh, my great-grandfather. Jawala was in his early teens when he returned to Kot Khera after the British wars. He was a literary and religious man and owned 18 ¾ acres of land, most of it at the boundary of Shahpur village, about half a mile southeast of Kot Khera. The land was irrigated by rain and much later by a well.

---

[5] My brother, Surat, located and interviewed Manga Singh, a descendent of Jassa whose elders went from Kot Khera to their *jagir* in Mangowal but later settled in Khatkar Kalan, a village nearby. That village is the birthplace of Bhagat Singh, a famous freedom fighter, a terror to the British government, and a folkloric martyr.

After he died (thought to be anytime before 1914), his three sons, Inder Singh (my grandfather), Gurdit Singh, and Waryam Singh, inherited the land and divided it equally into three parcels of about six acres each. One went to the eldest, Inder, but it was not enough for the bare survival of his wife and six growing children aged seven to nineteen. The remaining 12 acres or so went to Gurdit and Waryam who lived as a joint family all their lives: the two men, their wives, and Gurdit's adolescent son, Amar. The land was enough for them to live comfortably.

Gurdit, Waryam, and their families were financially much better off and did not have a lot of warmth for Grandfather's family. They met only on social occasions. Gurdit's son, Amar, in turn had two sons, Beant and Sowarn, and a daughter whose name I cannot remember. Waryam, had no child of his own and adopted Beant as his heir.

My great grandfather's *haveli* was square in shape and covered an area of less than an acre. Grandfather's share was closest to the path leading to a nearby canal and was not walled off from the two-thirds that belonged to my granduncles. Grandfather's *haveli* was an empty shell enclosed by a wall on three sides in which there was one room and a few mangers. Grandfather also owned a small house in the center of the village.

The period up to 1914, or until the outbreak of the First World War, was very difficult for my grandfather. He worked alone on widely dispersed land patches to support his wife, five sons (Isher Singh, Kesar Singh—my father, Paul Singh, Jamer Singh, and Sohan Singh), and a daughter who died early in adolescence. This period of poverty was deeply engraved in my father's and uncles' memories, and it became a powerful motivating factor in their lives.

Chapter 2: My Life Begins

My Childhood (1922-1936)

I was born on May 12, 1922 in Wadala Khurd, Amritsar District of Punjab, in my mother's parents' house. Father had just graduated from a three-year academic course with the degree of Graduate of Punjab Veterinary College (GPVC) in Lahore.

Five years later, Father took me with him to Lyallpur where I began my schooling. Mother or Bibi as I called her, and my younger brother Makhan, who was born in 1925, were still with my grandparents. After a few months, Father and I moved from Lyallpur to the Veterinary Clinic at Dichkote where the rest of our family was to join us. It was March and still too cold to sleep in the open. Since the Veterinary Assistant (VA) whom Father was replacing had not yet vacated the official residence which we were to occupy, the hospital office became our makeshift home.

My first visual images are of my father studying his professional literature while I did my homework. Both of us would sit or lie on our beds with a kerosene lamp burning brightly on a table at the head of our beds. I was not quite five years old. Within a few days, Bibi came. She had her hands full with household chores and the day-to-day care of Makhan. A year later, my brother Surat was born. According to Bibi, I did not need much of her attention and did not suffer from sibling rivalry.

The Veterinary Hospital or clinic had a spacious square area enclosed by five-foot high walls, two side-by-side rooms with a patio in front, and two rooms at the back. One of the two front rooms served as an office while the other was used to store drugs and medicine. The two rooms at the back, also side by side, were a temporary animal shelter but were usually unoccupied. The VA's quarters were adjacent to the clinic.

Dichkote and My First School

My school was across the road from the clinic. It consisted of two sections that were joined back-to-back: primary grades one to four and secondary grades five to eight. There were striking contrasts between the two sections.

The primary school that I attended was at ground level and built out of mud. It looked decrepit when compared to the red-bricked secondary school which sat at a higher level and was much more impressive. In the primary, we squatted on jute carpets which were laid out on the floor and held our reading or writing materials on our laps. In the secondary school, students sat on wooden benches with desks. Getting to the secondary school was my goal in those early days.

Writing lessons also illustrated the resource gap between the grade levels. In the secondary school, and this is what delighted me most, students used paper to write on with nibbed pens dipped in blue or black-blue ink bought from the store. However, in the primary, math questions were written with soft slate pencils on wood-framed rock slates that could be wiped clean. Dictation was written with a reed pen on a *phatti* (small wooden board). The *phatti* was thin with a smooth surface, a handle, and measured about 18" by 14" in size. Once its both sides were full of writing, it would be washed off and a thin coat of inexpensive yellow clay reapplied to its surface. This was allowed to dry and then both surfaces would be lined with a lead pencil. The board was thus ready for another writing session and lasted the primary years. India ink crystals were dissolved in water and were quite suitable for writing. Our pens were made from reed stems. These relatively cheap writing materials and the absence of school fees made primary education within everybody's reach, but it was not legally compulsory.

One day while Father was rummaging through old books and records in his medicine room, he came across two registers that were mostly blank, except for a few pages of written information of no real relevance to the clinic. He was ready to throw them out, but when I asked, he gave them to me. I was fascinated with these registers. I could write in them with my pen, and in a few days, I had them full with my school work!

The four grades of primary education in those days stretched over five years, since the first grade required two years of schooling; the first year was called "the soft first" (*kachi pehli*), and the second year was "the solid first" grade (*pucci pehli*). Annual examinations for all classes up to grade ten were held in April.

In Dichkote, I had complete freedom to roam around on my own, and I took full advantage of it. During my two years' stay, I explored most of Dichkote and its surroundings. The state of security in our community was such that neither I nor my father ever had any worries. Like most children, I was observant and very curious. I used much of my after-school hours watching what Father was doing. When I asked, he would explain to me, as if I were an adult.

One of the many interesting cases that I recall was when I saw him shoot a horse that was suffering from Glanders in one of the rooms used for housing indoor patients. He then buried it in a deep pit under the floor with a thick layer of limestone all around. He patiently explained to me that the animal had a disease that was highly communicable and fatal to humans, and that was why it had to be killed and the owner compensated, according to government law. The pit had to be at a place where there was no chance of it ever being dug up. (Its skeleton is probably still there today.)

A Frightening Incident

When I was six years old, I sat on Father's chest as he was lying down on his bed. We were engaged in a mutual playful teasing when I pulled his beard too hard. He threw me against the bedroom wall and into unconsciousness. As I regained consciousness, I saw with my eyes half closed that I was on his lap with my head resting on his left shoulder. He was in tears and urging me to inhale pungent vapors from lumps of ammonium hydroxide in a bottle. He intermittently brought the mouth of the bottle to my nostrils and took it back to give it a good shake. Withholding my breath while he had the bottle in front of my nose and breathing only when it was taken away, I continued to fake unconsciousness. After three or four minutes, Father started crying loudly, probably thinking that I was dead. I stopped faking. I had no injury that I could feel, but this terribly abusive act of my father became fixed in my memory. After that, I was always very careful when I was around him.

Another incident of Father's violent rage happened in Dichkote in 1929 when Father's Deputy Superintendent showed up at the clinic one morning, unannounced, for his annual inspection. He first watched Father treat the animals, but there were too many patients, and he could not find the time to conduct the inspection. He then asked Father to bring the registers to the resthouse where he was staying. Later, when they met, the superintendent became annoyed with Father and apparently threw the official clinic records in his face. Father then closed the door and beat him up, leaving him with a few bruises. The local police did not bring charges since the bruises were slight and there were no witnesses. Soon after, Father was served with transfer orders to Jatoyi, a small town in western Punjab close to Baluchistan, known to remain isolated during summer due to flooding of the River Indus.

This incident was a harbinger of serious changes in our family's life, since Father, on receiving his transfer order, refused to go and took a short casual leave, followed by six months of medical leave. I was sent to live with my grandmother and uncles in Kot Khera. Bibi and my two brothers went to live with my grandparents. This was only the beginning of Father's long list of difficulties.

Chapter 3: My Parents

My Mother, Bibi (1905-1965)

Bibi had a quiet disposition, subdued nature, and laissez-faire attitude. She was born in Wadala Khurd, Amritsar District and was named Ganga Devi after the sacred River Ganges, and commonly called "Gango." Her date of birth was not known even to her. In the India of those days, a date of birth or any other occasion hardly made any mark in the lives of poor people. They were mainly preoccupied with surviving the day-to-day struggle against starvation. Mother came from such a family.

She was the second child in a family of ten; her one and only brother was the ninth. A Brahmin family that lived next door during her childhood strongly influenced her life. She never ate meat, fish, or eggs in her life and, as far as I am aware, practiced *ahimsa* (avoiding all forms of violence to animal life) all the way in thought and deed. For many years, when we could afford it, she offered the ceremonial feast to a Brahmin, a holy or pious man, inviting him home during the annual Hindu festival of "Sharad." She believed in the segregation of the Untouchables.

Bibi was a beautiful petite woman of about five feet four inches with a round face, brown eyes, and jet black hair. Her forehead was narrowed from side to side by encroaching hair growth and one upper incisor remained visible even with her lips closed. She had a prominent scar on her left eyebrow from a wound inflicted in childhood when she fell from a tree swing while high in the air after one of the ropes broke. The three facial features added charm to her attractive and carefree face.

I was 13 years old when I realized how hard Bibi worked. Almost every day, she ground wheat into flour using a manual grindstone to make our chapattis. She plucked mustard greens from cultivated fields, simmered lentils, and milked our cows. She would chop mangos to make our year's supply of pickle. She processed and spun cotton for our sheets and quilts and washed, spun, and knitted sheep's wool into sweaters. They were coarse, but warm. She sewed and handwashed our clothes with her own brand of homemade soap. She kept my three brothers, my sister, and me clean, warm, and well-fed. She told us fairy tales, sang nursery rhymes, and lulled us to sleep many nights. She gave us love, made us laugh, and taught us right from wrong.

In early February 1965, my brother Surat wrote to me in Canada that he had taken mother to the General Hospital in Amritsar, suffering from abdominal pain. Following a misdiagnosis, she underwent a surgical procedure that revealed inoperable cancer of the liver. Surat brought her back to Kot Khera.

I immediately started making travel arrangements. But, only a week after receiving Surat's letter, a second letter arrived, announcing Mother's death on February 13. I was devastated. Bibi had been much more than a mother to me. She had shaped my life and the lives of my children. She had given so much of herself without ever asking for or expecting anything back. She was the only person I could talk to with an open heart. I will always remember Bibi's often-repeated compassionate statement when she was alone with me: "Son, you were only a teenager when you became a beast of burden with family worries." Her death opened a floodgate of grief and emotions. The trauma of not having seen Bibi during the most difficult period of her life left painful memories.

Father (1895-1982)

My father, Kesar Singh, was the second of five brothers. There is some evidence that he was born in 1895. He was about 5' 10" and very muscular with broad shoulders. He had prominent cheekbones, hollow cheeks, and a strong jowl. His wide ample forehead, brown eyes, and dark complexion reminded me of Grandmother. He became bald and grey in his forties and regularly colored his beard with henna.

Father was a powerhouse. He often rode his bicycle for miles on dirt roads with someone sitting on the handlebars and another behind on the carrier. He could swim across the Chenab River, which in places reached one and a half miles in width. He was only afraid of crocodiles. According to him, he was a good wrestler in his teenage years. He rarely drank alcohol and never smoked. He was jovial, had a good sense of humour, and a commanding voice.

A Soldier in WWI

My father, like Uncle Sohan, graduated grade eight from Khalsa School in Tarsikka. He was recruited for cavalry training around 1912. Uncle Isher, who was good at telling military jokes, probably played a role in my father joining the army.

Father was sent to the Second Indian Division (or Brigade), which was made up of one British and three Indian battalions. The battalions landed in Basra, Iraq, to reinforce the First Indian Division that had already captured Basra on November 21, 1914, and Shatt-al-Arab, the joint estuary of Euphrates, Tigris, and Karun Rivers. The southern region of Mesopotamia, or modern Iraq, was a vast land of river valleys with no roads or railways.

On May 31 of that year, Indian and British troops left their base at Al Qurna and assaulted Al Amarah, 87 miles away. It is highly likely that Father was with these troops. Major General Sir Charles Townshend was in command. Heavy shelling scattered the Turk defenders. After capturing Al Amarah, Townshend and his men set off in pursuit up the Tigris River with a fleet of paddle steamers and ancient barges. Arab villagers along the way waved white flags as the flotilla passed. Barges full of Turkish troops were captured as their officers cut them adrift from their steamers to beat a hasty retreat. The "Townshend Regatta" swept through Mosul and Qal-at-Salih all along the Tigris River banks (Townshend, 1920).

On August 20, 1915, the forces in which Father was serving were assembled at Al Amarah into the famous Sixth Division. According to accounts written in the *Encyclopædia Britannica*, this division performed miracles before finally surrendering in Kut. From Ali al Gharbi, Townshend with nearly 11,000 troops and 30 guns, launched a march along the Tigris in temperatures of 110-120°F. He was assisted by four flying reconnaissance planes. The objective, Kut-el-Amara, 153 river miles to the north, was captured on September 29, 1915, after Turkish front lines quickly fell and the Turks withdrew.

Townshend continued his advance toward Baghdad despite inadequate supplies, no proper plan, primitive communications, and insufficient troops to face the much larger Turkish force (Evans, 1935). He met with Turkish resistance at Ctesiphon, about 20 miles from Baghdad on November 22, 1915. The high river banks minimized the supportive effect of firing from the flotilla, and the Turks had shot down his reconnaissance planes. Indo-British troops suffered 4,000 casualties and a defeat. Townshend and his Sixth Division retreated to Kut on December 3, 1915. Four days later, the Turks laid siege to the town. Townshend had 10,000 men (including my father),

2,000 ill and wounded and 3,500 non-combatant Indians in his command. In addition, there were 6,000 Arabs to feed.

During the next five months, the Turks repeatedly attacked Townshend's garrison and repelled liberating forces from outside. On January 20, the annual floods from the melting snow of the Zagros mountains swelled the Tigris River, putting the Mesopotamia Plain under water. Kut was flooded and completely isolated. Scurvy, starvation, malaria, gastroenteritis, and dysentery claimed hundreds of lives. During the siege, 1,025 men were killed or died, 2,446 wounded, and 721 died from disease (Moberly, 1924). The final liberation effort, called "Dujaila Redoubt," was doomed and suffered heavy losses.

Father described the battlefield to me as a noisy place with putrid smoke from exploding shells and bullets and cannonballs shooting in every direction, strewn with wounded, mutilated, bloating, and dead bodies. Fear of death was constant, like a Damocles sword always hanging overhead. They often suffered from insomnia and nightmares. During the five-month siege at Kut-el-Amara, conditions were even more stressful. He and his fellow soldiers had to eat horse meat and cooked shoes and saddles. The garrison was bivouacked and poorly fortified, deprived of any active defense, and bombarded constantly by the Turkish artillery.

Father told me about a time when shallow flood waters caught him and others asleep. They had to spend the rest of the night sitting in cold water, not knowing in which direction to go. The next morning, Father said, he had a hard time standing up but, somehow, waded to the beach where he met an Arab woman who took him home and fed him dates.

Townshend finally surrendered on April 29, 1916 to Turkish Commander Khalil who sent General Townshend, alone, to Constantinople for captivity on an island in the Marmara Sea; 420 British officers were shipped to Baghdad, and from there to Anatolia in Turkey; and 10,000 Indian soldiers marched overland to a desert camp at nearby Shumran where they were flogged, raped, tortured, and starved as prisoners of war. (Over 6,000 soldiers died in captivity.) Of the 1,450 sick and wounded, mostly Indian soldiers, 1,136 were sent to Basra in exchange for Turkish prisoners of war.[6] Father

[6] The Mesopotamia River campaign began in October 1914 and ended on March 11, 1917 with the Turkish army routed and Baghdad in British possession. For details, see Cruttwell (1934), *Encyclopædia Britannica (1962),* Terraine (1965), Gilbert (1970), and Burg (1998).

was among the sick and wounded in this exchange. According to Father, his ordeal came to an end with the ending of the siege. He was lucky to escape being interned in Shumran as a prisoner of war.

Shell Shock or Schizophrenia?

Many soldiers who returned from the First World War suffered from "shell shock." The symptoms were highly variable and occurred as neurasthenia, anxiety neurosis, strong fears, obsession phobia, verbal outbursts, violent temper, and schizophrenia.[7] By the end of World War I, as many as one million cases of shell shock may have occurred. Two years after the Armistice, 65,000 ex-servicemen were drawing disability pensions for neurasthenia (Holden, 1998). More pensions were granted by the British Government for psychotic illnesses in 1929 than had been granted immediately after the war (Michell, 1931). Thom (1943) noted that 24 years after the war, 58 percent of all patients being cared for at veterans' hospitals in the United States (68,000 men) were neuropsychiatric casualties of World War I.

In retrospect, the violent episode with Father in 1928 was my first observation of his behavioral disorder. When I analyzed his symptoms, I found that his disorder did not conform to a textbook description of any specific psychological disease. His insidious disorder worsened with age and evolved from, or consisted of, difficulty dealing with people who opposed him, a flawed perception of reality, depression, and continued insecurity. In addition to these symptoms, there were others which changed as he got older and occurred retrogressively in four stages.

The first stage, which I noticed when he was still young, was his unpredictable temperament. While he was mostly easy going, at times even minor opposition could precipitate a mild to violent response. He would fly into a rage and be ready for a fistfight, regardless of the consequences.

The beating that resulted in my father's transfer was the second incident, and a third occurred in April 1930 when Father and I were traveling by bus to Havelie Bhadur Shah to visit his new clinic. On the return trip, Father got into an argument with a fellow traveler. The argument turned into a dispute, and Father beat him up. The incident had an alarming effect on me.

The second stage began during his middle age, in the 1930s. Father's

---

[7] Riese, 1929; Gibbs, 1920; Michell, 1931; Copp and Andrew, 1990.

violent behavior subsided somewhat, but he was still quick tempered. I was then eleven, and the frequent recipient of jabs, slaps, and disparaging epithets. When I turned sixteen, he hurled frequent insulting and humiliating remarks at me that left deep emotional scars. I was rebellious and headstrong, but Father overstepped the limits of discipline, meting out punishment out of rage and indignation, and in a proportion that was out of line with the offence. He humiliated and insulted his superiors, right or wrong, and had difficulty dealing with people. He always thought he was innocent and was being unjustly persecuted. I found it intriguing that in between his agitated moods, he was always sincere, affectionate, helpful, and easy going.

The third or verbal stage stretched from around 1940 until Bibi's death in 1965. Father always had an insatiable urge to talk. He would talk incessantly to owners when they visited the clinic, often lecturing on the course, cause, symptoms, treatment, and prognosis of their animals' diseases, showing them pictures from books. Occasionally, his overwhelming anxiety would trigger a loud monologue on different subjects. I was a favorite topic. He would harp on how much better off he would have been if he had not had children. The discourse, once started, would go on and on and on, even when no one was listening. He could be heard from a long distance, and Mother and I found this embarrassing. These discourses revealed his underlying insecurity, suspicion, worry, illogical thinking, delusions of persecution, and a shrinking perception of reality. Surprisingly, his physical health did not suffer, and he was able to function at professional and social levels until after Mother's death, which triggered the final stage.

In the final stage, Father was overwhelmed with grief at Bibi's death. It disrupted the remainder of his life, and he closed his practice. He developed persistent delusions of being poisoned by the very family he loved and who loved him. His reasoning gave way to stubborn hallucinations, for which he vehemently refused all treatment.

He began to wander off. Once, he was found in Hardwar, a pilgrims' city on the Ganges River in northern India where Hindus and less commonly Sikhs go to bathe in the holy water for salvation; another time he went to Amritsar's "Gaowshala," a charitable cow sanctuary funded by public donations; he was also found in Pinglewara, an institution for seriously dysfunctional amputees in Amritsar and in Amritsar's Golden Temple complex.

Toward the end of the 1960s, his condition became a full-blown disorder.

I worried about whether the disorder might be caused by genetic factors but was somewhat relieved that, as far as I was aware, none of our descendants had ever had similar symptoms. It was hard to exclude the traumatic effects of the war in Mesopotamia and the siege at Kut-el-Amara as a possible cause.

Father, a Veterinarian

The end of the First World War brought optimism and happiness to Father's life. He and Uncle Isher were home safe. Father entered Veterinary College in Lahore on a leave of absence with a commitment to return to cavalry service on completion of his studies.

In the 1920s, there was an economic depression of global dimension, the causes of which have never been fully clarified. Among the reasons frequently offered are that the rates of currency exchange and trade flow between countries were unrealistic and unevenly balanced so as to benefit France and the United States, which had acquired most of the world's gold (55% by 1929). Other countries, in an effort to conserve whatever gold stocks they had, raised interest rates high enough to discourage speculators from changing their investments into gold. Since the world operated on the gold standard, all countries required gold reserves to back up their paper currency. There was high consumer borrowing, shrinking economic growth, and widespread unemployment. These effects became worse in India due to the heavy debt left from the First World War, and for several years, the government of Punjab deducted 10 percent from the gross salaries of all public employees for what was called the "War Fund." The Indian government further tightened its belt by demobilizing troops.

After completing his studies, Father was discharged with a monthly pension of five rupees and remained unemployed for almost two years. He served as a veterinarian for about a year at Pak Pattan (now in West Punjab). Soon after, he was interviewed in Lahore for the job of veterinary assistant (VA) to the Director of Veterinary Services. At the end of the interview, Father asked the director's personal assistant and office superintendent (PA) about his chances of getting the job. He answered the question with a question:

"Do you make ghee (clarified butter free of impurities) in excess of your needs, since being a farmer, you must have cows?"

Father, getting the cue, returned a few days later with about 36 pounds of ghee in a sealed metal container (pipa). The next day, he was given the letter appointing him reserve veterinary assistant at Layallpur Veterinary Hospital. After nine months of probation at Layallpur, he was confirmed and transferred as VA in charge of the Veterinary Clinic at Dichkote.

Punjab's Veterinary Department

Until 1947, Punjab had been a large province that included Pakistan's Punjab (West Punjab), India's Punjab (East Punjab), most or all of the newly created Himachal Pradesh and Haryana Prant Provinces, but not the six erstwhile states – Patiala, Malarkotla, Kapurthala, Nabha, Jind, and Faridkot – then ruled by rajahs or maharajahs. The Province of Punjab had a chief of veterinary services designated director, and below him were eight superintendents, one for each of the province's divisions. Under them were 24 deputy superintendents, one for each of the province's 24 districts. The province also had a veterinary college and an animal breeding farm. Each district had many veterinary assistants (sometimes also called veterinary assistant surgeon depending on the educational standard), each in charge of a veterinary hospital or clinic. There was generally one clinic in a ten to fifteen mile radius, depending upon the animal population. Each clinic had three more employees: a dispenser or pharmacist who mixed drugs according to the VA's prescriptions and two helpers who restrained the animals during treatment and kept the clinic's premises clean.

The Veterinary Department's main concern was the treatment and prevention of illness in agricultural and domestic animals. A veterinary assistant provided treatment for sickness in the clinic and vaccination of healthy animals in the villages. All these services were free of charge. A VA was only allowed to charge a fee when he attended sick animals at their owners' residence (house calls), and this only when not on duty at the clinic.

Father told me about his trouble with the deputy superintendent during his annual inspection of the clinic in 1929. He had asked Father to bring the hospital registers and other records to the resthouse or *Dak* bungalow where he was staying. *Dak* bungalows in northern India were government-owned buildings that were maintained by the provincial public works department for the convenience of government officers touring the area on official duty. They were available for a nominal charge and were generally located at the outskirts of a city or a major town. They consisted of three to four rooms, a flower garden, and a surrounding wall. They had a caretaker and, sometimes, a cook.

The incident with the deputy superintendent had occurred because there had been no gifts or payments. Father had, therefore, undermined his traditional authority. Father's assault was difficult to understand and might have been due to excessive pride getting in the way of judgment. In laying the blame for this dispute and its aftermath, it is essential to place this event in the right perspective and to know the mitigating circumstances. In those days, it was an ongoing custom for animal owners to pay a small fee when their animals were either treated at the clinic or vaccinated in the village. Owners had a misperception that treatment and vaccination were not free, and if they were, then the quality of the service must be inferior. Hospital staff promoted this perception by being cold or indifferent toward owners who were unwilling to pay, and this discouraged many owners from coming to the clinic. Though unlawful, the fees collected by hospital employees were usually divided on a pro rata basis among themselves, with the VA getting the lion's share. A few disallowed or discontinued the acceptance of such illicit fees and only accepted charges for the customarily allowed house calls.

I believe that the practice was no secret to the deputy superintendents or the superintendent. A vast majority of them and their deputies approved and even encouraged it so they could receive their share. Some of them had devised cunning means of harassment and intimidation. I am convinced that the value and frequency of the offerings, in addition to flattery and obedience, were important criteria in a VA being promoted to deputy and then to superintendent.

Paying tribute was a centuries old tradition in Indian society. Under Hindu rule and later under Muslim emperors, *assignment* was a distinctive institution in which most of the country's land was assigned to rajahs and chieftains. The tradition was alive and flourishing during Father's tenure as veterinarian and was still widely prevalent in 1952 when I myself worked as a veterinary assistant surgeon.

In 1934, while Father was working at Jahania Mandi, a deputy superintendent made a surprise visit to his clinic. Father had been overworked and was behind in his recordkeeping since he did not think that it was a pressing matter. In those days, hospital records were maintained in three registers: outdoor patients, medicine, and vaccine. The outdoor register contained the owner's name, diagnosis, drugs administered, and, at the end of each day, the total of all drugs expended. The last item had to be carried over every day to the medicine register for an updated individual balance of all drugs in the clinic. If verified on any given day, the balance of each drug in the register had to equal quantity on hand. The deputies were known to calculate the balance of drugs and measure or weigh drugs to find discrepancies. In the vaccine register, a VA recorded the owner's name, number of animals vaccinated, the total vaccine used, quantity in stock, and details on animals. Since the vaccine was available free from the Veterinary Department and had no commercial value, it was unlikely to be misappropriated. A deputy might sometimes be so thorough as to go to the extreme of verifying the number of animals and their owner's name as given in the vaccine register.

I watched while the deputy checked the written records and noted several discrepancies. He then checked the average daily attendance of patients (an indicator of Father's popularity in the area) and questioned animal owners regarding his effectiveness. He invited complaints from owners and checked the hospital rooms and premises for cleanliness. I found this inspection to be far more exigent than some of the later ones made by superintendents. Ironically, they were quite often satisfied when Father was eager to please and willingly provided all the food for their and their orderly's stay, which would be about three days. (All these expenses were, of course, officially paid by the department.)

In the months following the inspection, the deputy kept firing off letters, generally in English and occasionally in Urdu, asking for explanations and threatening Father with disciplinary action. Following departmental policy, copies of all the correspondence, including Father's explanations, would be sent to the superintendent and the Director of the Punjab Veterinary Department thus influencing their opinions. A copy was also filed in Father's personal records to counter weigh any future promotion. The method of annual assessment in vogue had nothing to do with Father's professional competence or his usefulness to the people.

As a result of the inspection, Father was punished with a transfer first to Multan for two months, then to Mailsi for another two months, and finally to Rangpur – yet another isolated area ravaged by summer floods. The scenario with Father refusing to pay tribute or submit in servitude, the ensuing harsh inspection reports, and transfers to remote villages became a hallmark of my father's service record with the Veterinary Department. I witnessed events like these repeatedly.

Father, a Dedicated Professional

From his first day in charge of a veterinary clinic, Father neither accepted nor allowed any of the clinic's employees to accept illegitimate fees. He assured owners that they would get quality service as their due right, and it soon became clear to them that his primary focus was the welfare of their animals. He examined every animal himself with genuine interest and personally gave all treatments – drenching, injections, and surgery. His positive attitude, pleasant temperament, and humorous anecdotes became well known. His charm and professional competence inspired confidence and kept owners coming back again and again. Wherever he was posted, daily attendance increased four and five-fold. His kindness earned him much affection, and owners thanked him over and over for having made a difference in the lives of their animals and, in turn, in their own lives.

While in Rangpur, an area of widespread poverty, Father hardly ever charged a visiting fee to which he was entitled and, yet, rarely refused to see a sick animal at its owner's residence. During this period, he served the poorest of the poor. Quite often, a farmer who had walked to his clinic would get a ride home on the back seat of Father's bicycle, for anywhere up to ten miles on a dirt road, in addition to a free-of-charge visit. If the owner who needed his help lived in a village which was closer by swimming directly across the river than by taking the ferry, he and the owner would swim side by side both ways with their clothes tied in a bundle on their head. The river, during monsoon rains, could be up to two miles wide with strong mid-stream currents.

Once, on my way home for the summer holidays, I took a bus from Multan to the end of the bus route. As I had arrived too late in the afternoon to safely walk the last ten to twelve miles to the ferry, I was directed to the headman of the village for help. When I mentioned Father's name, he gave me a warm reception, an excellent meal, and a comfortable overnight stay. The next morning, I had a camel to ride to the ferry and an attendant to bring the camel back. All the benefit of my father's reputation.

A Miracle Cure for Sciatica

At the end of May 1941, Father was admitted to the Multan General Hospital suffering from sciatica. He went on extended sick leave and eventually recovered. In the summer of 1943, Father's sciatica pain recurred, only this time it was worse. He was confined to bed with excruciating pain that could only be relieved temporarily with hot compresses all along the sciatica nerve, from hip to ankle. We heard through the grapevine about a "savant" (or *sianna*) who lived in a village off the Jallo Railway Station (near Lahore). My brother, Makhan, and I took Father to see him.

The village was quite big and not too far from the railway station. We learned later that it had been founded a long time ago by a gentleman whose family name, by a strange coincidence, was Khera. He had two wives: one Muslim, and the other Sikh. The descendants of his Muslim wife continued in the Muslim faith, and those of his Sikh wife in the Sikh religion. Thus, about half of the population of the village was Muslim, and the other half was Sikh. The *sianna* himself was Muslim and one of the headmen of the village.

Throughout our journey, which was in part by *tonga* (two-wheel horse-drawn vehicle) and part by train, Makhan and I virtually carried Father on our backs. He had not been able to stand up on his own, let alone walk for about a month. When we reached the village, our *tonga* driver let us off at a large area shaded by bunyan trees with many cots laid out. This was where farmers socialized during the noon hour when the sun was too hot. We laid Father on one of the cots, and I went to the village to fetch the *sianna*. His wife told me that he was working on his farm and that she would send someone for him. We were to wait under the bunyan trees. A while later, a tall handsome man in his early forties came and introduced himself. What followed next was incredible.

Father related to him the history of his disease. He then asked Father to touch the areas that were painful. Father couldn't because all the pain had disappeared. He asked Father to stand up, and Father stood up; he asked Father to walk, and Father walked; when he asked Father to run, Father ran for about twenty yards. Then, with a sharp blade, the *sianna* made three intersecting superficial cuts covering an area about the size of a large coin in the skin above both hips. To this area, which seemed to correspond with the origin of the sciatic nerve, he applied a grey powder. He instructed us to wash the wound with soap and lukewarm water and anoint it with *ghee* every day, adding that the wound would heal in about three weeks. He then left without accepting any money. We were later told that people came to him from near and far to be treated for sciatica, and he never charged a penny. Father never felt sciatica pain again.

Father retired on June 15, 1957 after serving nearly 31 years in 18 different towns and villages. His starting monthly salary was Rs60. When he retired, he was earning a mere Rs135. Thereafter, he had his own practice until shortly after Bibi's death.

While I was in Canada, over a period of nine years, my family took care of Father in Ludhiana off and on. All this time, he resisted treatment and was entirely out of touch with reality. In 1975, he moved to Bareilly with my brother Surat and his family. Surat kept me informed of his health through frequent letters. His psychoses worsened, and he trusted no one, firmly believing that everyone was trying to poison him. In 1982, he choked on food, developed pneumonia, and died on February 13 after a brief illness. My mother had died on that same day 17 years earlier.

From his modest beginnings, my father became a highly respected veterinarian. He dodged the frightening paranoia for most of his life, but eventually it overpowered him, rendering him totally dependent on his family. Sadly, his honesty made him a victim of tyrannical corruption and oppression by unscrupulous bosses. He inspired, encouraged, and nurtured a love for learning in me and my children and, thus, shaped our lives. Despite his faults, which I am convinced were due to his insidious illness, I always loved and respected him.

Chapter 4: Life in Kot Khera

My Dadi Ji (Grandmother)

My grandmother, Attar Kaur, was my surrogate mother twice: the first time for seven months when I was seven years old and in second grade, and the second time for six months when I was around eight or nine years old.

Dadi Ji came from a poor farming family of Dhilwan in Amritsar District. She was a soft-spoken, petite, caring, and compassionate woman. She was very popular among the neighborhood housewives. They would come to visit and talk to her about financial, marital, or other problems. She would listen patiently and, from time to time, nod her head in sympathy. She was an extremely loving mother figure, radiating a warmth that made me feel comfortable and secure. I never seemed to miss my mother when I was living with her. I have fond memories of her lovingly calling me "Duddyai," which means a small or young frog.

Dadi Ji lived in the village house with three of my uncles – Isher, Paul, and Jamer. Uncle Sohan had been posted to Amritsar. The house had two small rooms and a high wall made of mud that enclosed a small area in front. One of its corners was designated as a kitchen. It had a primitive firebox, warded off on three sides with mud walls to retain heat and open on top for a kettle or pot and in front for adding wood or dried cow dung cakes. The rooms were lit with kerosene oil lamps. Dadi Ji slept in one room while I slept in the second with one of my uncles. My other two uncles slept in the *haveli* to watch over the animals. The trio took turns exchanging the two sleeping places. During the hot summer, we slept on the roof.

I recall that in the summer of 1938 Dadi Ji was suffering from acute sciatica of both legs and was utterly dependent on Uncle Jamer, who was always there to help her when she needed him. Nobody even tried to get her treated because, in those days, a disease followed its own course, and medical treatment was a privilege for those few who had money.

Later on, the two-room house in the village became too small for all my uncles, two aunts (one with a baby born in the early 1930s), and Dadi Ji, so they moved to the *haveli* by the mid 1930s, making it their sole residence.

During my first stay with Dadi Ji, two events stand out in my memory: the construction of a new building for the primary school and Uncle Sohan's wedding.

Granduncle Waryam Singh

While with my grandmother, I frequently saw my granduncle, Waryam Singh, riding his small, playful, and lively mare in an outward display of horsemanship. When not riding, he could be seen in the company of his beautiful wife, Bishan Kaur or Bisi as she was called. Bisi had one of her dimpled cheeks tattooed with a lentil-sized round mark to enhance her beautiful face. Theirs was an ideal marriage, as if they were custom fit for each other. They often walked together, and they were always more than willing to talk to anyone about the latest gossip or share a joke. His wife had a rich vocabulary of folksy proverbs and would come up with one most appropriate to the occasion. Their conversation was always unhurried and engaging; both were good at talking and listening, but better at the former.

Granduncle was about 5' 6", had a fair complexion, slim body, short neck, Roman nose, and relatively prominent cheek bones. Auntie was about the same height and complexion. Unless we ran into them by accident, they stayed aloof from our family, and we never developed a meaningful relationship. Even with others, their personal relations were casual and neutral, as was their non-confrontational attitude toward many affairs affecting village occupants. They did not make many friends, nor did they make enemies.

Judging from some of the historical events that occurred in his lifetime, Granduncle was about 80 years old in 1960, and his wife was not too far behind. They both enjoyed excellent health then, but Granduncle was slightly hard of hearing. He had a poise and pride that was endearing to me. They were satisfied with their lot and didn't want for anything more.

Our *Haveli*

Uncle Isher Singh had joined the army in 1908 and trained in the Indian Cavalry. Before going to the Franco-German war front in 1914, he came home on leave and handed over his savings to Grandfather. With this money, Grandfather bought red bricks to renovate the old *haveli* and add new buildings. Most of the labor must have been put in by my grandfather, Uncle Isher, 23, and my father who could have been 19 then. Paul was still an adolescent whereas Jamer and Sohan were too young to be of much help. The project consisted of erecting two rooms, one at the back, the other in front, and a new wall facing the entrance to replace the old mud wall.

The new brick entrance or front wall was higher and rather impressive. It had a solid wooden gate that was big enough to let in a large bullock-driven cart. There was a small window on one side of the gate that could be opened from inside or outside just big enough for a person to squeeze through without letting the animals escape. On the left side of the gate, they built a spacious room with its floor elevated from the ground perhaps with the mud left over from the room before. The room had two doors, a window on each of its two walls and a built-in safe for cash with a locked wooden door. The new room was large enough to accommodate the male members of the family and guests who would sleep there during the winter or when it rained. During the summer they slept on the roof.

At the back of the *haveli*, stretching across its entire width which was about one-third of its length, were two rooms of the same size, one in front of the other. They were linked by two doors. The wall of the front room facing the gate was built out of bricks and had three equally spaced doors. These, as well as the gate, had turned silver grey from weathering and appeared to have been especially made of well-patterned wood pieces assembled with great skill. The front room was used for sleeping and living by my aunts, their children, or my aunt's parents when they came to visit.

Facing each end of the front room was a kitchen area with a firebox marked off by a mud wall. Occupying the middle area on both sides was a long manger that had several wooden pegs in the floor to which the animals were tethered. The area on the left between the front and back rooms (upon entering the gate) had a roof to protect the kitchen and the animals from the elements. On the right, inside the gate, was a hand-operated water pump, a square brick surfaced area for bathing, and a tamarind tree for shade. All in all, our *haveli* was one of the better ones in the village.

The toilet, as for all the people in the village, was anywhere outdoors in the nearby fields before daybreak and, later in the day, among the waist-high crops; water for cleaning oneself had to be carried along in a receptacle.

In 1916 or early 1917, Grandfather slipped off the roof and died from his injuries. After his death, the economic survival of the family became all the more precarious because the army wages of Isher and my father were meagre, whereas Paul, 12, Jamer, 10, and Sohan, 7, were not yet ready for farm labor.

There was not enough land for any worthwhile contractual income. In those days, even for the hardiest, there were extremely limited opportunities to make a living. Having a half-decent meal on the table was a big treat. The poor lived for food and starved when there was none.

My Uncles

My two uncles, Paul and Sohan, their wives, the remaining two bachelor uncles, Isher and Jamer, and Dadi Ji all lived as one family sharing land, work, income, and home. Sohan looked after accounts receivable and payable, while Isher made all the important decisions for the family, in consultation with all members. They got along with each other exceptionally well and made an excellent team. Their single goal was to break the stranglehold of poverty that had loomed large for decades.

Farming was a dawn-to-dusk, seven-day-a-week operation using only primitive implements powered by muscular strength and stamina. There was hardly any time for social activity or entertainment. Ploughing an acre of land took two men four to five hours, each walking about 16 to 18 miles. Ploughing was tediously slow because the plough had only one iron blade or plough share to cut six-inch wide furrows. It was pulled by a team of yoked oxen, with the men holding the oxen's nose string in one hand while the other maintained a steady pressure on the handle to keep the blade deep in the soil. Irrigation was even slower and would take two pairs of oxen two days to irrigate an acre of land with well water. The family weeded with a hoe and picked cotton and threshed cereals by hand. They would cut fodder with a sickle, bundle it, and carry the bundles on their head.

The agricultural methods in use then had not changed much over the last 30 centuries. Somewhat similar implements and methods were reportedly being used much earlier than the birth of Buddha, during the Rigvedic Age, estimated to be about 1200 B.C., and in the region around the south of the present Ambala (Berriedale, 1962). Interestingly, the area is less than a hundred miles from Kot Khera.

With no chemical fertilizers, pesticides, or herbicides, crop yields were poor, and the price of cash crops (cotton and wheat) was low. High quality wheat in a market favorable to a farmer sold for about 1½ rupees per 40 kg.

My uncles had saved enough money to buy large tracts of land. They turned their poverty into prosperity with hard work, thrift, and trust in each other. They shared the value system which was forged out of their struggle.

They had integrity, strength of character, respect for human dignity, and a positive outlook on life. They minded their own business and never had trouble with the law. My aunts, Phinon and Dhanon, though, were reluctant to share their husbands' aspirations, since they found it difficult to live in perpetual denial and sacrifice. However, they had no choice.

They never forgot how Grandfather's early demise had left the five fledging brothers to fend for themselves and struggle for their survival. Their shared hardships, efforts, and accomplishments became a strong unifying cement that held them and their families together. The strong brotherhood ties were an example frequently cited in the village where even a minor incident between brothers could split families apart forever.

Their diet was simple: home-grown leafy vegetables, lentils, beans, yogurt, and flatbread made from wheat and corn flour. Meat was limited to very special occasions. They did not use tobacco, alcohol, or the readily available marijuana which grew wild.

They all dressed alike: they wore a muslin turban, closely fitting *kacha* (a type of Bermuda shorts) and, during winter, a *chaddar* loosely wrapped around their legs and tied at the waist. Except for the turban, all these garments were white and made from home-grown and homespun cotton weaved from coarse yarn by our village weaver. Their shoes were made of thick, tanned leather and lasted at least one and a half to two years.

Since my three younger uncles were orphaned in childhood and forced to work on the farm for a living, they did not have access to education. They were brought up in a society with very limited opportunities. They attributed their lot in life to their karma in a previous life. They had a deep faith in reincarnation and never questioned its validity. They grew up understanding life in simple terms and accepted it more because of their faith than for any other reason.

Uncle Isher Singh

There is no firm information as to when Uncle Isher was born, but it could have been in 1891. He may not have stayed at school long enough to read and write well. In 1908, he enlisted in the Indian Cavalry and was dispatched to the war front in the Franco-German zone. At the end of the war in 1920, he was demobilized with a monthly pension of five rupees and spent the rest of his life farming at Kot Khera until his death in January 1979.

After Grandfather's death, Uncle Isher, being the eldest, became a father figure to his brothers. He excelled in hardiness and endurance: there were accounts told that, in 1934, he had brought home on foot a small herd of cattle from 250 miles away, and then, a year later, a young female camel from 300 miles away. Impressive feats! His life on the battlefront had made him callous and impervious to sympathy, compassion, even love.

While I was visiting the *haveli* in 1938, I noticed a photograph on the wall of our living-bedroom; it was the only decoration in the room. I asked Uncle Isher about it, and he went on to give a glowing account of his battlefield achievements, adding with pride that the photograph had been taken in Paris. Later on, I again asked him about Paris. What had impressed him most about the city? He awkwardly fumbled and groped to find a suitable description. He appeared to be having difficulty bringing back to memory a visit that not only had been brief but was 20 years old. With some hesitancy, he enumerated two things: honesty and that the streets had been made of glass. He then told me that he had forgotten his wallet in a pub one night and that someone had returned it to him the next day. As to the glass streets, he was partly right since I remembered from my time in Paris in the 1950s seeing small areas of thick glass in places, probably to light up the underground tunnels.

He never married, and his income from the pension and small piece of land should have been sufficient for him to live an easy life like my granduncle Waryam. However, he chose to work hard for no other reason than to make a better life for his brothers, particularly Sohan and his children. He got along especially well with Sohan and always took his side, right or wrong, as if bonded to him.

Uncle Paul Singh

I would guess that his date of birth may have been 1900. I'm not certain that he could read, write, or even sign his name because I never saw him do any of these. He became head of the family at age 15 when his father died and his two older brothers went to war.

He was unique in several ways. He was soft-spoken, unassuming, and rarely said anything that might hurt anyone's feelings. He was one of those rare persons who never got angry. He seemed content and happy, had no particular ambition, nor was he interested in novelty of any kind, not even travel. As far as I can remember, he left the village only twice: once to go to Wadala Khurd for his own wedding and a second time to go to Amritsar for a court appearance in a land dispute. His silent and bland temperament was often the flip side of his emotional strength and stability.

He was slim, tall, handsome, and graceful. He hated to make decisions, even those affecting his immediate family. For example, even the marriage and education of his children were mostly decided by his more assertive younger brother, Sohan.

Uncle was married to Phinon, Mother's sister. He had two sons and a daughter. The oldest son, Kartar, was born in the early 1930s. He had blue eyes like Uncle Sohan and was very handsome in his youth, but had little energy, freshness, or fire. He failed the pre-medical course (Faculty of Science Diploma) twice, married in July 1950 and again a few years later, quit farming to drive trucks in Delhi and, at last count, was somewhere in southern India.

On our trip to Kot Khera in March 1990, my wife Claire and I briefly visited my uncle's second son, and, by chance, his sister was there. She was very warm and kept insisting that we go to see her husband and family at their farm in nearby Tarsikka. We could not go because the area was then infested with terrorists. Our host (cousin) was very loving and his wife even more so. They entertained us with tea and eggs. It was Claire's first visit to a *haveli*.

Uncle Jamer Singh

I have fond memories of Uncle Jamer when I went to stay with Dadi Ji. He took me along whenever I wanted to accompany him, and he answered all my questions in seriousness. Thanks to him, I experienced the childhood thrill of sleeping overnight in fields that were being irrigated with slow moving well water and among mounds of harvested wheat. I was supposed to help him guard against thieves.

Also thanks to him, I got to see the extraction of oil from mustard seeds: the seeds were ground into a fine powder in a huge cup-shaped wooden mortar by the crushing action of a club-shaped wooden pestle rotated in a circle around the mortar by an ox. The extraction of oil was a cottage industry which disappeared in the 1930s. He took me to the village shoemaker who made shoes from home-tanned hides which, unless softened by several oil applications, caused painful blisters above the heel. I got to meet the village goldsmith and watched him make rings from gold. Uncle Jamer also taught me how to keep a herd of cattle grazing on a pasture *without* fences. This was least exciting of all since it required a lot of running to bring back errant animals every time they left the pasture.

Uncle Jamer had no formal schooling but had learned how to read and write in Punjabi on his own. He was fond of books on religion, history, and the politics of Sikhs, which he frequently discussed with his brothers when they were working together. He was five feet seven inches tall, had pleasing facial features, and a finely chiselled nose.

I spent much of my time away from school with Uncle Jamer. He was the warmest, most affectionate, and compassionate of all my uncles. Perhaps he acquired these feelings from Dadi Ji, the same as he had inherited her deep brown eyes, dark complexion, and facial features.

Uncle Sohan Singh

Uncle Sohan was born in 1908, had grade eight education from the neighboring Khalsa School in Tarsikka, and was a constable with the Punjab Police Department. I recall his wedding vividly. It was the summer of 1929. Mother had become quite a matchmaker since she arranged for him to marry her sister, Dhanon. She had also arranged Uncle Paul and Phinon's marriage.

According to custom, the wedding ceremony was held at the house of the bride's parents. Uncle Sohan had invited all his relatives, including myself, and some 30 friends. We formed a wedding party and traveled on horseback to Wadala Khurd, the bride's village. At the outskirts of Wadala, the party was met by a band of musicians that had been hired by Uncle Sohan. They played drums, flutes, and clarinets, making sure to catch all the villagers' attention. The music was characteristic and auspicious of the impending wedding. On hearing the music, shaggy-haired villagers in bare feet and ragged clothes came rushing to meet us.

I rode in the procession behind Granduncle Waryam on his mare, which is my earliest recollection of him. He stayed in my memory most probably because he would frighten his nervous mare, and me, every time he popped up his short body straight from the stirrups to gain the necessary height to lob coins over the heads of the people in front. As was the custom, Granduncle, like others in the procession, repeatedly threw fistfuls of coins to the poor. The crowd created a scene, fighting, yelling, grabbing, snatching coins from each other, and falling down in an effort to maximize their prize of copper coins.

Soat was a common practice then: members of the wedding party would preface the happy beginning of a wedding with a display of charity by throwing large quantities of coins to the poor of the bride's village. The event was ironic in two ways: the wedding party would get the credit for the charitable act when, in fact, all the coins had actually been provided by the bridegroom. It was a poignant contrast of the snobbery of some and the indignity of others. It offended me. S*oat* was eventually replaced by a custom in which the bridegroom gave money to the bride's father who would then distribute it to the poor of the village. Later this custom, too, was abolished.

Chapter 5: A Tumultuous Childhood

On the Train Alone

In December 1929, Father was appointed as reserve veterinarian at Jhang Maghiana after his six-month medical leave. I said goodbye to Dadi Ji and went to live with Father in a spare room on the hospital premises, while the rest of our family remained in Kot Khera. He was on probation at the veterinary clinic preparing for his test while I attended grade two. We were together most of the time, studying in the night, going for our meals to a *dhaba*, a roadside eatery. Once, we even went to see a silent movie in a circus-like canvas tent. This was my first movie and quite a treat.

In April, Father and I took the train to bring our family from Kot to Havelie Bahadur Shah, Father's new posting. We got off at Amritsar to change trains. Father left me with my suitcase and blanket in the next train, which was due to leave in about half an hour, and went to buy our tickets for the rest of the journey. The train started to move, and Father was not back yet. It was just before sunrise, and the light was dim. It didn't bother me that the train was leaving and Father was not back. I had the presence of mind to recall that I had to get off the train at Jandiala Guru to go to our village. (The town was named after the tree known as Jandi under which a guru lived and prayed; it was later changed to Jandiala.) When the train first stopped, I looked out at the name on the station, which was not where I had to get off. When I spotted the name of Jandiala on the next station, I took my suitcase and blanket and got off the train.

I crossed the overhead bridge to the main railway station. Feeling sleepy, I made myself a bed by laying the blanket on the ground and used the suitcase as my pillow. A short while later, a man came up to me and asked me my name. When I told him, he identified himself as the stationmaster and informed me that he had received a message from Amritsar railway station that my father had missed the train and was on his way by bus to meet me here at the railway station. Father later told me that he had missed the train due to long line-ups at the ticket counter. He was surprised to find me calmly waiting for him without any worry; after all I was only eight years old.

After a few days, we collected our family and returned to Havelie. The clinic and residences were in the wilderness among mounds of ruins. The place was eerie and spooky at night. Our home was about a mile from the village, and I had to walk along a lonely path through agricultural fields and wasteland to reach my school. From the very first grade, I had developed an interest in fiction and loved to read stories of black magic, miracles, witchcraft, and ghosts. They fascinated me, and my fascination was probably stimulated by the strangeness of the area in which we lived. Curiosity drove me to watch for long periods of time the calving and the newborn calf's struggle to walk and nurse, the chameleon on an acacia tree changing color, the male camel in rut, too angry to be loaded with burden.

With avid interest, I would watch our pharmacist going through the lengthy process of converting arsenic into a powder that he claimed had aphrodisiac properties, properties I didn't understand then. He would carefully pack the arsenic into a hollowed-out branch of a pomegranate tree and place it in the fire. He would recover the packed piece after it had been in the fire for a day and night. The process, known as making *kusta* was the center piece of quackery imported to India long ago. Starter materials, such as gold and jewels, were said to have even greater aphrodisiac effects than those of arsenic. Evidently, these claimants would not have gone out of business had this been true.

Seven months after our arrival, Father was implicated in a lawsuit. Bibi, Makhan, and Surat went back to Wadala, and Uncle Jamer came and took me back to Kot where I stayed with my beloved Dadi Ji and uncles and passed grade three in the new schoolhouse. Father was acquitted in the lawsuit and was posted to Jahania Mandi, a small town in Multan Division. In May 1931, Bibi, Makhan, Surat, and I, escorted by Uncle Jamer, traveled by overnight train to join him. Our family stayed in Jahania Mandi for three years. My sister, Darshan, was born there in 1932, and a brother also named Darshan was born a year later.

The Division was populated immediately after the First World War when its network of canal irrigation was first established to make farming a profitable venture. The Punjab government awarded land free of charge to First World War veterans who pledged to raise and sell mules and thoroughbred colts to the Indian army or to those who planted large tracts of trees and nurtured them. Whatever land was left was auctioned off at bargain prices to be paid for, interest free, over several years. The rural areas produced lots of wheat and cotton that could be traded in the many markets of Multan Division. Jahania Mandi was one of them, and its name, literally translated "world market," was appropriate.

My First Academic Achievement

All schools in Punjab were on the same schedule; classes began in April and ended with an annual examination in March. The first year was considered pre-school level in preparation for academic studies at age six. These included Urdu, mathematics, geometry, history, and geography. English and another language, Punjabi or Persian, were added in grade five, and science was studied in grade nine. The curriculum for all schools across the province up to grade ten was the same, as were the text books, which had to be approved by the provincial school board. A change of school anywhere in Punjab would hardly make any difference to a student. The schools emphasized security, discipline, and learning. Teachers were figures of authority, inspiration, and hard work. They had patience, time, and interest in the welfare of students. We respected them just as much as we respected our parents.

When I was in grade four, the head teacher at our school announced that he would be selecting two students to go to Khanewal High School for a scholarship competition in which selected fourth graders of the District competed. I was elated when he selected me and a fellow classmate out of a class of about 40 students. I felt proud of myself. I succeeded in passing the test, although not in winning the scholarship. But I felt very special, indeed, at having stood first, in aggregated marks of all subjects combined, in grades four, five, and six with a class size of about 30 to 40 students.

Father and I at Odds

Growing up, I had been a sweet little boy who would run up and do whatever my father would ask me to do. Around the age of 11, I began asserting myself with a newly developed feeling of self-confidence, which my father would not accept. He absolutely refused to cooperate with me. He kept demanding that I run errands or fetch whatever he needed and expected immediate and total compliance! Some of his demands were too frequent for my convenience or came at inappropriate times when I was playing, reading, or doing homework. Any delay, reluctance, or refusal would upset him. Father would then slap my face or jab me and call me with my new name *kamla* (insane), quite often in the presence of owners of sick animals in the clinic. I resented the treatment and felt deeply hurt and insulted.

Once after my brother, Darshan, was born, Bibi had made a big container of sweets for herself so she could get her strength back. She kept them under lock and key, but I knew where the key was, and I stole a little bit every day. One day she caught me and raised a big commotion. Father heard from the adjoining room, came in, and gave me a jab or two and a stern warning to stay away from the sweets.

During that year and the first half of the next, there were several isolated confrontations between Father and I, but two of them were particularly contentious and lingered over most of this period: Father's bicycle and my soccer game.

Father had bought a new bicycle, and he rode it quite often. Like any child, I, too, wanted to ride it. When I asked him to help me learn, he not only flatly refused, he also told me in clear terms to stay away from his bike. It was summer, and Father used to sleep a couple of hours in the afternoon after closing his clinic. He always kept the bicycle in the house, close to the door. While he napped, I would sneak out his bike to learn how to ride on my own. It was an adult bicycle, and when I sat on it, my legs couldn't reach the pedals. I devised an alternative method. With my left foot on the left pedal, I would run the bike forward, and as it gathered speed, I would pass my right leg through the frame and onto the pedal. In this position, the bicycle and my body were slightly tilted toward the ground. Learning to pedal, get up a good speed, and at the same time maintain my balance was a difficult and slow process. I fell down frequently in the beginning, but less and less as time went by, thus raising my hopes that the pleasure of riding was within my reach.

After about an hour's practice each day, I would meticulously clean off all the dirt and dust from the frame and put the bike back exactly where I had taken it. The arrangement worked well for a long time until Father woke up earlier than usual one day and failed to find the bicycle in its usual place. On my return, Father greeted me with a couple of jabs and a warning never to touch his bicycle again. From then on, I was more cautious and would take out the bicycle only when father was out-of-town!

An Introduction to Soccer

The Veterinary Hospital, the dispensers' house, and our house occupied two end-units in a complex of ten single-story brick units built in a straight line with an end-to-end roofed gallery in front. The last unit at the opposite end was the residence and office of a postmaster, who had a son, Jagat Singh, about my age who was also in grade seven. His parents gave him a soccer ball as a present. One day, he told me that his toes hurt because he didn't know how to kick the ball properly, but he was keen to learn. I eagerly showed him how to kick the ball barefoot using the middle upper part of the foot while tightly pulling back all the toes at the time of impact. He was impressed by my expertise and anxious to learn all about my past experience, which I was not at all reluctant to share with him.

I had been introduced to soccer a few months earlier by a well-known player named Rashid who was home for the summer holidays from Islamia College, Lahore. He was a graceful player who later became very famous, despite having a malformed arm and hand. He had brought a soccer ball with him and was staying with his father in a house directly across from ours. There was an open dirt field in between. His father, a butcher and meat shop owner, always sought the goodwill of my father who, in addition to his VA duties, inspected live animals and meat for human consumption for a small honorarium from the municipality.

One day I saw Rashid in the open field all dressed in a uniform and soccer shoes running around aimlessly chasing his ball. Anxious to make friends, I introduced myself and expressed interest in playing with him. Probably aware of the connection between our fathers, he was very courteous and taught me how to kick, dribble, and pass the ball.

Soon, we were kicking from opposite ends toward a makeshift goal. The game was more tiring for me since after his one kick at the goal I had to kick several times to get the ball back to him. Rashid was happy that I was sparing him the trouble of running all the way back to fetch the ball, and I was happy to hear frequently that I had the makings of a good player. From time to time, we both would be running after the ball for possession and control. Rashid was about 20 years old, and I was 11. Soccer was all that we had in common.

As far as soccer was concerned, Father had tolerated it well so far, though he was not very happy with my toes which were receiving daily sessions of long soakings in cold water. The soccer practices continued for two to three months until Rashid returned to college. When I told Jagat about Rashid, he wasted no time in organizing ten of our schoolmates to play soccer on a daily basis in a field at the back of our complex. Our soccer field was a barren tract of land with side boundaries approximately defined by imaginary lines drawn between surrounding bushes, with a goal on each side of the field marked by temporary goal posts.

Since none of us were familiar with the game, we invented our own style and rules, which we modified as time went by. The game, in essence, was to snatch the ball away from an opponent and run with it until it was either lost to an opponent or kicked at the goal or, when totally out of breath, passed on to a teammate as a last resort. Quite often such passes were interpreted as signs of generosity and true sportsmanship rather than strategy. From our own experience, we had developed a short list of fouls expedient to playing without too many interruptions. Shoving and tripping were not only acceptable but even encouraged for their general appeal to all of us and also because it made the game more challenging. In all matters of dispute and setting game standards, Jagat's word was final because he owned the ball and made no bones about reminding us as often as he could.

Two fouls that everyone agreed were serious were fist fights and violently pulling the opponent by his clothes. Fighting could cause hard feelings; plus, we ran the risk of losing a player. Pulling clothes generally tore the only clothes that most of us owned. Obviously some of us, overly mindful of physical appearance, did not want to be seen in rags. Also, our mothers were very inquisitive and would not take on the mending unless explanations were forthcoming as to what, who, why, and not again after you promised it wouldn't happen again and other related cross examinations were satisfactory to them. Quite often the details were so unpleasant that we would rather forget than repeat them.

Sometimes, when I would mention my soccer games, Father would quietly listen, alert me as to possible physical injuries, and show a sort of indifference. I translated these as signs of encouragement. In a few days, our soccer game expanded to socializing. Previously, we used to go home as soon as our game ended when it was too dark to play. But now, we would squat after the game and engage in conversation on topics of common interest – teachers, parents, or current gossip. We would then bathe in a small canal nearby, and by the time I would get home, it would be about an hour and a half after sunset.

After a couple of warnings, Father imposed a curfew; I now had to be home within an hour of sunset, and failing that, there would be no evening meal. The sanctions did not work. I would sneak in the kitchen when everybody was sleeping and help myself to the leftovers. Frustrated in his efforts, Father declared one day that if I came back after the curfew, I would not be admitted into the house. It was September, and the nights were cool where we were living.

The next day, as I was about to leave for my usual soccer game, my younger brother, Makhan, asked me if he could also come to play. (My other younger brother, Surat, was too young to stand up to the rigors of our brand of soccer.) We were always looking for more players, and so I took him along. After the soccer game, we had our social chat and canal bath, as always. When we reached the house, there was no light, and all the doors were locked. The front gallery had a wooden chair and a bench where clinic clients waited. Makhan and I took the bench and the chair in turn; one of us tried sleeping on the bench while the other sat on the chair waiting his turn. The next day, Makhan refused to accompany me, saying that what he had experienced the night before was not his idea of having fun. For a few days after that, I came home on time. Very soon afterwards, the soccer ball started losing air pressure, probably a spur from one of the acacia trees surrounding the field had punctured the bladder. When we tried to reinflate it, the rubber bladder burst beyond repair. Sadly, our sport had come to a sudden end.

Induction into Veterinary Politics

In grade seven, I was quickly inducted into veterinary politics at the age of twelve. Father asked me if we could both put our heads together and come up with a reasonable explanation for his deputy's queries. Father was not quite fluent in English, the preferred language for official correspondence. Although I was just learning English, my writing was clear, which was important to his correspondence; as time went by and my education advanced, I became his ghostwriter, taking over all his correspondence.

My earliest lobbying mission for Father came when I was 14 years old and a boarding student in grade nine at the government school in Khanewal. On my way back to school from Rangpur, where Father was posted, I stopped at Deputy Kahn Singh's house in Muzaffar Garh, a district city, to deliver two large baskets of mangos. These were from our rented mango garden that produced much more than we could eat. The deputy was on the verge of retirement and on friendly terms with my father. He invited me in and treated me with civility and warmth, which was normally the way that adolescents were treated by their elders.

On several occasions, Father asked me to lobby or campaign on his behalf when he was in trouble with his superiors, unfortunately a common occurrence, and act as an emissary or messenger of goodwill when he was at peace with them. This was because Father could not be absent from the clinic without approval, and getting such leave was a lengthy process.

In the middle of September, my parents decided that I would return to school at Jahania Mandi to continue grade seven and stay in its boarding house. They put me on a bus from Mailsi to Multan, which dropped me off at a railway crossing about three miles from Mandi. It was a hot summer day, and I walked on a deserted path along the railway tracks carrying a pack weighing about 25 pounds, full of books, clothes, and bedding. I had to stop many times to rest, as the pack was very heavy. I passed by the soccer field and canal, where I used to play and bathe. I met no one until I reached the fringe of town, yet I was not afraid.

After a month in school, Father came for me, and we joined the rest of our family who were waiting in Multan. We then proceeded to his new clinic in Rangpur. Rangpur has been romanticized by the poet Warris Shah in his famous love story of Hir Ranjha. The town is located on the shore of a large river that flows from the merger of the Jhelum and Chenab Rivers. The route to Rangpur was time consuming, difficult, and quite often strenuous because of flooding. From June to October it could only be reached from Multan by bus to its terminus, then by foot, horse, or camel for about ten to twelve miles to a ferry station, and finally across the river by ferry. For the rest of the year, there was a convenient train or bus ride of about 18 miles from Multan to Muzzafar Garh, and from there to Rangpur by bus.

Postal service during the summer was irregular, since the village remained isolated by river floods. All around Rangpur for miles, there were date trees growing wild loaded with fruit during the summer. There were also mango trees everywhere. If anybody wanted to eat, all he had to do was climb up a tree and help himself. During the summer, it was common to see dates drying in the sun, spread out on mats made of date leaves in temporary enclosures fenced in by similarly made mats. Exporting dates was a profitable local industry.

In grade eight, the headmaster, Pairra Ram, and my English teacher, Ram Lal, were very devoted and hard working. Ram Lal taught us translation of short descriptive essays from Urdu to English and how to write concise narrative essays in English. I developed writing skills in Urdu, which was the main language in school. Urdu, a word of Turkish origin, was given to a language written in Persian script with a vocabulary derived from Arabic, Persian, Turkish, and Hindi languages. It was used in rudimentary form by Muslim rulers and their armies until the 17th century, when Muslim seminaries in Delhi and Lukhnow developed it into a literary language. In my time, Urdu was taught as a starting language in primary schools in keeping with the purported wishes of Punjab's ethnic majority, whose mother tongue paradoxically was Punjabi. After India's independence, Urdu was replaced by Punjabi and Hindi in East Punjab.

We were taught Indian history, geography, mathematics, geometry, elementary civics, political science, and an additional language, Persian or Punjabi. A student wanting to pass grade eight had the choice of taking an examination conducted either by his or her own local school or by the divisional school board in each of the eight divisions of Punjab Province. The examination was difficult, competitive, and rewarding. A few students at the top got a two-year scholarship. All candidates were administered standard tests with the same questions, which were not the type that required short responses or selection from multiple choices. They needed moderately lengthy answers. The answer books were coded and marked for test scores by different examiners in a process that tried to maintain as much uniformity as possible. A candidate was measured against students from other division schools with a standard scale of comparison. I took the examination at Muzzafar Garh with at least a few thousand other students. I was fifth in the division and won a scholarship. I was admitted to grade nine at the Government High School at Khanewal in April 1936 and stayed in its boarding school.

From 1934 on, Father had stopped hitting me, except for a single incident when he slapped me out of frustration. It was during the summer of 1934, and we were attending the annual picnic. There was a lunch of chapattis, vegetables, and sweets, followed by swimming and frolicking in the water. Most of the people of Rangpur were there. After a while, Father took me to the river with the intention of teaching me how to swim. He tried to make me float while supporting me with his hands. As soon as he removed his hands, I would sink. This went on for a while, but then he got frustrated with my failure to float. He slapped me across the face and left me in the river. (I finally overcame my fear of the water and learned how to swim at age 78.)

At the end of that summer, I started spending most of my time after school and during holidays playing a game that resembled field hockey with my schoolmates. It was played with an old tennis ball and tree branches that we shaped like hockey sticks. The time spent with Father was reduced to a few hours a week. I would see him at lunch time, which was, in many instances, used up by diatribes, such as: "You are spending too much time out of the house; I doubt your friends are doing you much good." I felt uncomfortable in his company, and our relationship was not improving. This was when I turned to Bibi for comfort and assurance. But Bibi was extremely busy with my one-year-old baby brother, Darshan, two-year old sister, Darshan, Surat who had just started going to school, and Makhan who was a second grader. With all the household chores, there was little time left for me.

Chapter 6: My Wedding

My Betrothals

Marriages were always arranged by parents in those days. The girl's parents would search, often for a long time, to find a boy they liked. They would then approach his parents for approval. Betrothal, a brief ceremony, took place at the boy's house and was attended by the boy's family, the girl's father, and the religious priest. The girl, who was about to become engaged, remained on the sidelines during the entire process. The wedding would then take place anytime that was suitable to both sets of parents.

The earlier practice of killing girl babies resulted in a female-to-male ratio of seven to ten in the farming communities of Punjab. This gave a girl's parents a lot of choice in finding a suitable match. That was the reason two of my uncles remained bachelors. The two who did marry had Bibi to thank, for she had arranged for them to marry her sisters, with my maternal grandparents readily agreeing to weddings without dowries. This was undoubtedly very much on the minds of my father and uncles as I was the next available bachelor at the age of nine. In retrospect, I find this an unfortunate irony since, in our society, the custom of child marriages (or betrothals) had long ago disappeared.

I faintly recall a man, probably my would-be fiancé's father, who came to see me at school and asked many personal questions. I remember telling him that my father was in government service and that I planned to continue my education. My responses presumably were a great plus in my qualifying the pre-betrothal test. And so, toward the end of my stay at Kot, I was betrothed to a girl whom I had never met or heard of before. Uncle Jamer had written to Father about the betrothal, and my father had agreed to it in a return letter. All I knew was that the girl was about my age and lived with her parents in a village of Amritsar District.

As was the custom, a representative of her parents brought a *kuja* missary (a circular mass of crystallized cane sugar about five inches in diameter), *parna* (a piece of coarse cloth about the size of a bath towel), and a few *showhara* (jumbo dates). These dates are symbolic of the betrothal ceremony, which itself is called *showhara*. Uncle Jamer had told me that all the items would be mine at the conclusion of the ceremony. They were all laid out in front of the beds on which members of my family sat. The village priest from our *gurdwara* began the ceremony by reciting a lengthy prayer. My mind, though, was on the *kuja* missary and *showhara* and on the good time I would have eating them. At the end of the ceremony, the priest, in keeping with tradition, told me that I now had a girl waiting to marry me any time my father wished it. Uncle Jamer gave me all the goodies, which I thoroughly enjoyed for a day or two.

In the summer of 1933, Father received a letter saying that the girl I was engaged to marry had died. So, at age eleven, I was again an eligible bachelor, a status that was short lived. A few days later, Bibi told me that the next morning I should be on my best behavior, since a lady was expected at our house. If she approved of me, she would become my mother-in-law.

When I got up in the morning, I heard Bibi talking to a visitor in the kitchen. They were having *chah* (tea). When I entered, the visitor gave me a quick head-to-toe look as if checking me out for defects. Afterwards, my future mother-in-law asked me a few questions, probably to make sure that my mental faculties were in order. Several days later, the betrothal meeting took place at our house. There was no priest or ceremony this time, and I didn't get any goodies, which was rather disappointing. I was again promised in marriage, this time to Rajinder, who later became my wife. I remember, though, that Father and his friends got drunk, and he was sick all night since he was not used to drinking alcohol. That was the only time I ever saw my father imbibe.

Joy and Grief on the Same Day

From the time that I was engaged, Father was under intense pressure to set a wedding date through letters and even a special visit by Bahadur Singh Bal, my future father-in-law who promised to look after Rajinder until I became independent. Finally, Father agreed and the wedding date was set for June 15, 1937, about a month after I turned 15.

Rajinder's parents had migrated from Sathiala in the District of Amritsar to the village of Chak 153/10R, which was about ten miles from Jahania Mandi. Her father was affectionately and appropriately called Shalungi (meaning small and thin). He was compact of body, had formidable energy and stamina, and worked for his wife's brother, Bhan Singh. By sheer luck, Bhan had acquired during the First World War two large canal-irrigated chunks of land, about twelve miles apart: one of 100 acres and the other of 450 acres. By the late 1920s, most of this land was under cultivation, and the remainder was being reclaimed from bushes and small trees, thanks to Shalungi's single handed efforts. In return, Bhan made him a gift of 25 acres.

Bhan was the biggest landlord in the area. His two sons and grandsons died young, as did his only daughter who would have been about Rajinder's age. He was Rajinder's godfather and had raised her from childhood. For all intents and purposes, he was her father. He was paying all of the wedding expenses, which was taking place at his residence in Chak 118/10R. Before the wedding, Bhan approached Father about the dowry. Speaking on my behalf, Father told him, "Your daughter is the only dowry my son would like to have."

Bibi bought fine cloth and hired a tailor who set up his operations at the house for several days to sew new clothes for the whole family. The floors and walls of the house were given a new layer of mud plaster. Bibi borrowed extra beds and bedding from neighbors to accommodate guests staying at our house. Uncles Jamer and Sohan from Kot and Bibi's brother, Sadhu Singh, and her father, Gurdit Singh (my only living grandfather), arrived from Wadala. Father had invited about 20 friends from neighboring villages to join the marriage procession on the ten-mile trip to Chak 118/10R. He had hired a bus and a band of musicians. The procession was set to leave in the afternoon.

Early in the morning, my brother Darshan suddenly developed a high fever. His dog and constant companion sat by his bed and would not touch the food in his bowl. The local doctor had no diagnosis but assured us that it was nothing serious. The procession went on as planned.

The next morning, just before the wedding ceremony, the officiating priest brought up two snags. The first was that Mother's family name, Sekhon, and that of my future wife, Bal, were closely related. This was readily resolved when he was told that the two families had not had a common ancestor for several generations. The second was that I was not baptized to Sikhism. Father promised that the baptism would take place soon after the wedding. (It never did.) With the problems resolved, the ceremony took place with our Holy Book, *Guru Granth*, in the midst of the congregation that included all the family members of the bride, her neighbors, and all the members of the marriage procession. Bibi had stayed home to minister to Darshan.

Rajinder was dressed in the traditional red *shalwar*, shirt, and veil, and I wore the traditional orange turban. The ceremony started with a lecture from the priest, which was essentially a list of dos and don'ts for the bride and bridegroom. I was unable to comprehend their importance, much less their significance. Following the lecture, the bride's veil was tied to a sheet (somewhat like a beach towel) which was wrapped around my shoulders. I then lead my bride-to-be around *Guru Granth* four times; each time we would pause and recite hymns from *Guru Granth* specifically written for religious weddings. The ceremony ended with the distribution of sweets made from cream of wheat, *ghee*, and sugar.

Father left quietly immediately after the ceremony. Nobody knew that he had gone, not even me. He never returned. All members of the party spent that day as guests of Bhan, who was an extremely hospitable and lavish host. The following afternoon, three days after our arrival, I brought my wife, her escort, and the remaining members of our party home.

When we arrived, we were shocked to learn that during our brief absence the family had been struck by a heart-wrenching catastrophe. Darshan had died. His sudden death came at about the time I was going through the wedding rituals. This, then, explained Father's sudden disappearance. As was the custom, Darshan had been cremated before sundown that same day. Bibi, tormented with grief, and Father, profoundly anguished, put up a brave face to welcome my bride to their house. I was stunned and in shock. I could not begin to imagine how my parents could cope with the simultaneous emotions of sorrow and joy evoked by Darshan's death and my wedding.

Following an age-old custom, Bibi welcomed my wife, her face still covered by a veil, and me by pouring ceremonial coconut oil on the door sill just before we entered the house. She then paid the ceremonial money in bills (*varna*) to my wife so that we could see her face for the first time. That night, Rajinder slept in a separate room with her escort. They left the next morning to go back to my in-laws. The wedding was over.

In the next few weeks, Darshan's dog howled continuously. He refused to eat and died, evidence of the unbreakable bond between them. Darshan had been the baby of the family. He was very handsome with brown curly hair. Bibi had nicknamed him *Bawa* after a curly-haired Holy Man, who occasionally came down to the Plains from his Temple in the Himalayas.

Chapter 7: Living Hand to Mouth

Harvest Time at Kot

Eventually, life returned to normal. I finished my grade ten in Khanewal and, at the end of March 1938, came home from boarding school. Father was constantly finding fault with me and was overly critical of everything I did. With only a few coins in my pocket, I ran away from home and hopped on a train to Kot Khera.

The train fare was not a problem. While studying in Khanewal, I had made friends with Krishan Lal, whose father was a guard with Northwestern Railways. Krishan knew all the tricks on how to travel without a ticket and had taught me well. I knew how to get in and out of railway stations, outwit ticket checkers, evade ticket collectors, and, if caught, solicit sympathy by saying the right things. Krishan and I had traveled to Lahore for the all-India exhibition of 1938 and back first-class without a ticket. I stopped this practice after I joined Veterinary College in 1948, but by then, I had been to places as far as Calcutta, Bombay, and Madras several times and had been caught only once by a ticket checker who was tenacious and would not settle for anything less than a breakfast. It had cost me all of four rupees.

I arrived at Kot just before the wheat harvest. Harvesting, in those days, began with a festival on Baisakhi, the first day of the Indian month Baisakh, which generally falls around April 13. Farming families from neighboring villages gathered on the fairgrounds for religious services, followed by lavish feasting, entertainment, and wrestling – kabbady, rope pulling, and volleyball contests. The harvest festival was similar to our Thanksgiving, except that it was celebrated before the harvest not its end.

The work was physically demanding, and my uncles had wheat maturing over large areas. They were glad to see me, since an extra pair of hands was always welcome. During the following month, I worked shoulder to shoulder with them, cutting wheat stalks at the root and tying them into roughly 32-pound bales with ropes that we twisted on the spot from wheat stalks. The bales would then be carried on our heads to a central area in the field and stacked one on top of the other in a 12-foot high semi-circle, five to six bales wide.

In front of the stack, a circle was drawn around a heavy post to which a pair of yoked bullocks was tied. They dragged a compact mass of acacia branches (*phallay*) over the stalks of wheat. The trampling and crushing action of the animal's hooves released the kernels from the husk and, at the same time, broke up the wheat stalks into fine straw that would be used for cattle feed. One of us had to walk around with a whip beside the bullocks, otherwise they would stop. As soon as the kernels were released, the kernel/straw mix would be raked into a pile close by and replaced by fresh wheat stalks from the stack of bales.

The whole process went on for several days until all the bales were transformed into huge piles of kernel/straw mix. The kernels would then be separated from the straw, bagged, and sent to market. The straw was stored in the *haveli*. During the entire process, we had to guard against theft and arson; I took my turn sleeping overnight among the piles. When the harvest ended, I was exhausted.

This experience taught me a valuable lesson – that poverty was a built-in feature of the agricultural economy. A farmer's future invariably depended on his past and his parents' past, since the size of inherited landholdings was determined by the number of offspring in his and previous generations. I saw farming as a dead-end, low-scale operation. The only way out, that I could see, was through education.

Once the harvest was over, Uncle Jamer took out his bike and a one rupee silver coin from the family's kitty. With me on the back seat of his bicycle, we set out on a two-day pilgrimage to the holy temple at Tarntaran, a 36 mile trip both ways.

The temple had an idyllic and graceful layout. The main g*urdwara*, an imposing marble edifice, sat like a majestic palace on an island in the middle of a huge, square swimming pool. The island was connected by a narrow path to a wide walking area (*parkarman*) that enclosed the entire pool. The *parkarman* was covered with square black and white marble tiles laid out in checkerboard pattern. Worshippers would walk into the temple, kneel, and touch their forehead on the ground in front of *Guru Granth* in devout supplication. Praying constantly, they bathed and walked around the *parkarman*. They could also sleep there if they wished. With time, the water level in the pool would become shallow, as silt from the canal water supplying the pool settled on the bottom. The pool then had to be emptied, and worshippers would dig out the silt.

At the end of the day, Uncle and I bathed in the pond and prostrated in front of *Guru Granth*. We ate our *prathas* with lentils cooked to dryness that we had brought from home and slept on the marble floor. The next morning, we headed home, stopping for a hot lunch at Aunt Moulo's in Dayew Bath. Uncle's one rupee was still intact! He told me that he had sincerely wanted to spend it but never really had the opportunity to do so.

Taking Responsibility for My Life

After I reached Kot Khera, Uncle Sohan wrote to Father, telling him of my sudden appearance there. Father had written back immediately asking me to return home – a request which I had been very reluctant to carry out. I finally went back toward the middle of May with one of Father's friends who had come to visit his relatives in a village nearby. Father was glad to see me.

Soon after my return, my parents asked me to bring Rajinder home. Bibi and Father were extremely happy to welcome Rajinder, and they liked her right away. We were both very naive and shy. We didn't know what to expect of each other. Father, Surat, and Makhan slept on the roof while Bibi, Rajinder, and I slept out on the patio. I think Bibi thought that I was still too young to consummate my marriage. However, in the middle of the first night, I got up and tiptoed over to Rajinder's bed and spent the rest of the night with her. The next night, Bibi took her bed up to the roof.

We enjoyed each other's company and liked sleeping together. She was tall, slim, and good looking. She had never been to school – there were none where she grew up – and had learned on her own to read and write in Punjabi. She sincerely and somewhat innocently believed in the dogmas, myths, and taboos of the Sikh religion. After ten days, she went back to her parents.

In the first week of June, I proceeded to Amritsar, where I was in first year at Khalsa College taking courses toward a Bachelor of Science degree in agriculture. The curriculum was tough and covered too many subjects. I boarded at Nabha Hostel, sharing a dormitory with three classmates. Soon, we became good friends. One of them, Manna Singh, played field hockey for the college and was selected to play on the All-India hockey team. He later joined the Indian army. I played soccer, but not very well. The remaining two roommates, Balwinder and Rashpal, were not interested in any field sports. Quite often, we played ball in the swimming pool and went to movies together. None of us took our studies seriously or did any homework. Picking up cues from each other, we thought that what we were doing was normal for college students. In the evenings, we would all sit together and talk about our aspirations and dreams for our future. Dreams were cheap then.

My roommates talked about their careers, fame, idealized love affairs, and happiness in its every conceivable form, to which I quietly listened. One evening, they asked about my dreams. I told them that I had been recently married. They were curious to know all about my marriage and seemed to feel sorry for me. After that, they treated me with sympathy as if I had lost one of my legs. I was impressionable and did not have much self-confidence. I thought that I was not entitled to share in their dreams and felt deprived of the love romanticized in fictions, drama, and poetry. As far as I was concerned, such love had become off-limits already at the tender age of 15. I was angry and resentful of my fate, which I thought was now sealed forever.

Exams were held in the month of March. By that time, I had lost all interest in learning, and knowing that I had no hope of passing, I quit college and came home in January 1939. I was a little apprehensive when I arrived, but once I explained why I had left, my parents seemed to understand and were not angry with me. In May of that year, under pressure from Father, I enrolled at Government College Multan. I attended classes for a month, but did not return after the summer holidays.

The next nine months were one of the most stressful periods of my life. There were three cyclical recurrences, each beginning with Father's long accusatory recounting of my past mistakes in humiliating language, followed by my running away. I was punishing myself with a vengeance. When my anger subsided, generally after two to three weeks, I would come back. Had my father, instead, tried persuasion and reassurance, I might have felt more secure and less resentful, but that was not Father's style. Better still, I might have been more understanding and less rebellious.

Father gave me his reasons for my early marriage. He said he did not want me to remain a bachelor, because a man needs to have a family. I remained unconvinced. By then, I knew that he wanted to control my life, and he had succeeded quite well. I thought I had to move on. Slowly, over those nine months, I came to realize that, whether I liked it or not, I had to take responsibility for my life and my wife, and the sooner I came to terms with my circumstances, the better it would be for the good of all my family. I was then able to start making the necessary changes.

With a renewed commitment, I entered the government college in Multan in April. Makhan and Surat attended the neighboring Dyanand Arya Vedic

(DAV) High School while Darshan went to the nearby primary school. We rented a house there, and Bibi came to live with us. This arrangement allowed us to continue our studies, since Father's salary could never cover boarding house expenses for the four of us.

I was energized by a new goal: to work hard toward a BSc degree and earn admission to Glancy Medical College, the only medical college in the Province of Punjab. My dream was to study medicine. In April 1941, I passed my first year, standing first in my class in zoology, botany, and chemistry (in a class of about 40 students) and obtained high marks in physics and English.

For the first time, Multan Division's Soccer Association sent a soccer team to Calcutta to compete in the All-India soccer tournament. I went as a substitute player, but ended up playing in both matches. The team left Multan in the middle of June 1941. Seeing a big city for the first time was very exciting. We lost in the very first match of the tournament and, on our way back, stopped to play a tournament at Patna. We then proceeded to Agra to see the Taj Mahal. Its white marble, majestic grandeur and glitter on a moonlit night was breathtaking. Its four symmetric minarets, each with stairs leading to the top balcony, were open to the public then. I sat on the balcony and enjoyed the panoramic view of the River Jamuna. I reached Kot Khera in the second week of July.

Back in 1934, while at Jahania Mandi, Father had been approached by a family in a nearby village who wanted to betroth their daughter, Banti, to Makhan. They promised to continue caring for the girl until Makhan had finished his education and became self-sufficient. Father had agreed. Now, her parents began putting increased pressure on Father for an immediate wedding. He finally consented, and Makhan was married in July 1941 at Banti's parents' house in a brief ceremony similar to mine. After their marriage, Banti continued to live with her parents.

Makhan had not wanted to get married. He even ran away the day before the wedding party was due to leave. But he was caught, and being a dependent, he had no choice other than to cede to Father's wishes. Father had succeeded in marrying his second son, despite strong opposition from all family members.

Amritsar: Nightlife with Rats

After summer vacation, our family unanimously decided to move to Amritsar so we could all continue our studies. Darshan was in middle school,

Surat in tenth grade at Khalsa School, Makhan in first year of college, and I in my second year. We rented a house in Putlighar, a developing community on the outskirts of Amritsar, 20 minutes walking distance from the school and college.

This was during the Second World War, when prices of all consumer goods, food, and clothing, in particular, were high. A family of six, like ours, with four growing members, needed at least Rs300 a month: Rs150 for food alone and another Rs150 for clothing, laundry, rent, transportation, etc. College and school fees added up to an additional Rs28 a month. Father's monthly income of Rs93 (75 from his pay plus 18 as inflationary allowance) fell far short of buying even the barest necessities of life. We made up the shortfall in part by selling milk and by bringing wheat and fodder from Kot to feed the animals. We had the clothes on our back and one change. Undershirts, underwear, and socks were luxury items. We had none.

When he was in Rangpur, Father had bought a young she-camel from a police auction of stray and unclaimed animals. Uncle Isher had brought her on foot all the way to Kot Khera, a distance of about 300 miles. Dachi, as we called her, was bred twice and gave us two handsome male camels. My uncles kept the two young camels and, reluctantly, allowed us to have our Dachi back. Dachi, a cow, and two buffalo cows were all the possessions that we took to our newly rented house in Amritsar.

The house was spacious for a small family. It had eight-foot high brick walls on three sides, two rooms and a built-in patio at the back, ample free area in front with a hand-operated water pump half-way between the patio and the front door. On one side of the patio, there was a stairway leading to the roof. With the first rainfall, we discovered that the roof leaked. Makhan and I had to carry on our heads large buckets of earth dug from nearby pits to give the roof a good slope for quick drainage.

A five-foot wide ditch ran all along the Ram Tirath Road which was on the same side as our house. It carried off drainage water and sewage and was a perfect breeding place for rats. Our house was lit with kerosene lamps. As soon as the lights were put out, the two rooms would turn into a playground for brown rats. They would come in either through gaps in the doorway or from holes in the floor, since the house was built right on the earth's surface. Repeated efforts to fill in the holes were readily defeated by the rats that proved to be very persistent, as if they thought they had just as much right to the use of the house as anyone else. A few attempts at using rat traps borrowed from our neighbors met with equal failure.

Our house reminded us of Karni Mata Temple which was built in the 17th century in the village of Deshnok in Bikaner (northwestern India) for the worship of rats. There, rats ran rampant and lived a good life eating coconuts and sweets. According to Hindu mythology, a rat was the constant companion of Ganesh (the elephant-headed god) and was considered to be the reincarnation of people hiding from the wrath of Yam (the Hindu god of death).

We had no such religious beliefs, but we had no choice but to learn to live with them. In the summer, the rats were less of a problem, since we slept outside. In the winter, though, we had to sleep with the quilt tucked in all around and under our bodies and heads, leaving only our noses exposed for breathing. The rats would crawl over the quilt, loll about, sit, and then scurry away. While feeling all their moves, I would go to sleep. I often still sleep with the blanket tucked in under and around me, leaving only my nose uncovered.

In May 1942, we moved into a neighboring house, which was in a complex named Bikhari Asthan, or beggar's haven, by its owner. The name came more out of a sense of humility than for any other reason. It had electricity and was built of red bricks, including its floor and roof. It had a row of three rooms. One was occupied by Bibi and Darshan. The door to their room did not shut properly, and so during the winter, the rats would come in through gaps in the doorway. Whenever my family came to visit, we had to sleep in this room. Rajinder did not like this at all.

The other room, the only one with a window, was occupied by Makhan, Surat, and me. This is where we slept (during the winter), ate, studied, and spent our leisure time. The middle or third room was used only in the winter to house our milch animals. Its open doorway was covered with a heavy curtain to keep the cold out. Part of the built-in patio in front of the rooms was used as a kitchen. There was a large spacious frontal area that was fully enclosed by walls and its entrance had a wide gate. During the warm weather, from April to mid-September, we slept in the open frontal area on beds that were covered by mosquito nets. We rented this house until August 1945.

Our Dachi

For about three years until 1944, Makhan and I walked with Dachi from Amritsar to Kot and back, a distance of 36 miles both ways, at least once a month and sometimes every weekend to bring fodder. We would struggle to load and unload Dachi with bales of clover cut from rented fields in a neighboring village. We also had to carry 40 kg bags of wheat on our heads to a flour mill that was about three-quarters of a mile from home.

Many interesting events occurred during our travels. Once, on the Grand Trunk Road to Kot, about three miles from Amritsar, we saw a very big guava garden, and the fruit was ripe. Makhan was hungry, and all the money we had between us was six pesas (about one and a half cents). Makhan entered the garden while I waited with Dachi on the roadside. A short while later, he came back with about 20 guavas. Makhan told me that when he had offered the garden owner all our money for some fruit, the man had told him that it was not enough to buy even one guava. Could he come up with more money? Makhan replied that he could not. Disappointed, he had started to walk away. The owner called him back and asked him to fold the front flap of his shirt into a sack, which he then filled with as many guavas as it could hold. Makhan told me that he was, indeed, very impressed with the owner's generosity and compassion.

Another time, we were stopped at Amritsar's Octroi Post (where duty was levied on goods entering the city) on Grand Trunk Road. Animal stealing was a common lucrative business then, and anyone traveling with animals was supposed to have a *Rahdari*. This was a letter written by the headman of the village where the animal's owner lived, describing the animal, giving the name of the accompanying traveler, and their destination. Written on an ordinary piece of paper without an official stamp, it did not even look like an official document. Also, the police did not have all the names of the headmen of every village in the province, nor the means to verify whether a particular signature was genuine. For these reasons, we had never bothered to get one for any of our travels.

When Makhan and I and our Dachi loaded with straw were stopped, we were asked to show our *Rahdari*. We quickly explained to the policeman that Dachi was ours and that we lived in Amritsar which, being a large city, had no headman. He got annoyed with us and took our explanation as an affront to his authority. He asked us to wait while he decided what to do with us. He returned to the investigation that he had been working on before we arrived at the post. After about two hours, he came back and authoritatively told us that he would let us go. I think that he had detained us without ever believing we were animal thieves. He had just needed to show off his authority.

For extra income, we sold all the milk from our cows and buffalo to our neighbors. Our diet was always the same: *chapatti* (flat bread made from wheat flour and water) and lentils or bean *dhal* (soup). Occasionally, Bibi would serve boiled *tori* (zucchini-like vegetable) that grew freely on the inside wall of our house. We were underfed and undernourished. Our food was low in protein, fat, and vitamins and was neither appetizing nor palatable.

Bibi had only one brother, Sadhu. I called him Mamoon Jan (meaning loving maternal uncle), partly in jest and partly out of respect. He was younger than me by six months. After he passed his matriculation in April 1942, Bibi suggested that he come and live with us so he could continue his studies at Khalsa College. I went to Wadala to invite him. He and my grandmother Gabo were extremely delighted with the offer, and so he moved in with us in the month of May. Now, we had one more mouth to feed.

Land Dispute at Kot

For at least 15 years, our uncles had cultivated our 12 acres of land and kept all the profits. When we moved to Amritsar, they agreed to give us half of the produce, which was then a customary return from tenant to landowner. Soon, though, they started sowing wheat in their land and fodder in all of ours. The wheat was a cash crop but fodder had no commercial value, and it was impossible for us to transport all of it to Amritsar. Our uncles had increased their income with wheat and at the same time ended up using up most of our fodder. We needed money, and this arrangement was unsatisfactory. We asked our uncles to stop cultivating our land so that we could rent it out. They started intimidating us and discouraged any prospective tenant-farmer from renting it. We were losing control over an important resource.

Father, Makhan, and I decided to go to Kot Khera to sort things out. We met with my uncles Isher and Jamer at Bagaiana Khuh. In the discussion that followed, Uncle Jamer was a passive spectator. Words turned to push, and push to shove. Uncle Isher attacked Father with a chopper, an 11" x 6" blade fitted with a handle that was used to cut the fodder. Before we could disarm him, he had made two gashes, one on Father's forehead, the other on my left hand at the base of the index finger. Neither was serious, but both Father and I were bleeding enough to alarm my uncles and to end the fight. The three of us set off for Tarsikka to obtain a medical certificate for bodily injuries and to press charges. The doctor was not expected until the next morning. We then went to the Veterinary Hospital to spend the night with Dr. Saini, a friend of Father's who was in charge of the hospital.

Within hours of the dispute, our uncles came with a *panchayat* of five influential members of our village who negotiated a deal that satisfied both sides. The final settlement, in return for not pressing judicial charges, consisted of full future cooperation by our uncles with anyone willing to cultivate our land, plus handing over the two young camels that Dachi had given birth to. Makhan and I walked home to Amritsar with the two camels.

A Humiliating Experience

At about the same time, a meat dehydration factory on a large tract of agricultural land in our neighborhood was nearing completion. The factory's enclosing wall bordered on Ram Tirath Road at its north and faced the agricultural farm of Khalsa College at its western perimeter. The factory operated 24 hours a day, seven days a week, slaughtering thousands of goats daily, slicing the meat into thin strips, which were then dried in hot compressed air. The dried strips kept well at room temperature and regained most of their original taste when soaked in water. All of the dried meat was sent to the battlefront to feed the Indian army.

The factory had several goat pens, and their water came from a network of channels that were linked to a well on the factory premises. The factory put out a tender to run the well twice a day for about an hour to fill up all the water channels. It was a well-paying contract and a rare opportunity to earn extra rupees. Makhan and I bid for the contract, thinking that one of our camels could be trained to pull water.

The well operated with a horizontal beam, with one end permanently fixed to a vertical rod while the other end was tied to one or two yoked animals. As the animal walked in a circle, it dragged the beam, which, in turn, rotated the rod. Through a set of gears, the rod turned a big wheel on top of the well, which pulled a chain with a series of metal jugs. These jugs would fill with water from the well and were then emptied in a large shallow flow-out chute.

Camels were often trained for many uses, and we had previously trained our Dachi for transportation with relative ease. With much enthusiasm, Makhan and I started breaking in our big camel at an abandoned well not too far from our house. This was strenuous work, and our camel had the required strength and stamina. During the next two weeks, our camel would run the well for an unpredictable length of time and then stop. We could not get it going again, as it would stubbornly resist every type of persuasion. Meanwhile, we got the contract and, hoping against hope, put the camel to work. Alas, it turned out to be a humiliating experience. Our camel refused to pull, and we lost the contract. We eventually sold both male camels for 850 rupees at the animal fair in Amritsar.

My First Paycheck

Throughout college, I had been receiving a monthly soccer stipend of seven rupees a month, which paid half of my tuition fees. I had to pay the remaining half before the fifth day of every month. In the spring of 1942, I couldn't come up with the fees in time; therefore, my name was struck from the college roll. I could not attend classes for two weeks until I was able to borrow enough money to pay the dues. Our financial situation was desperate.

In early 1943, an army captain (I do not recall his name), his wife, and two children rented the house next to ours. He had been assigned to the meat dehydration factory, to make sure that the factory operations complied with military specifications. His wife started buying milk from Bibi and soon became a good friend. The captain learned through his wife that we were struggling to get an education. He was very sympathetic. Wanting to help, he got me a job as chemist at the factory for the three months of summer holidays. I earned 60 rupees a month.

I wrote my final BSc examination with the practical test in organic chemistry on May 4, 1944. That same afternoon, the head of the newly created Rationing Department of Amritsar District interviewed about 60 candidates for five jobs – two enquiry officers and three assistant enquiry officers. I applied for assistant enquiry officer and landed the job of enquiry officer. For the interview, I wore a tie and ill-fitting coat, which I had borrowed from one of my friends who had been interviewed ahead of me. The very next day, I started working for 120 rupees a month pay.

I will always remember when I received my first paycheck. It was June 2, and my family and I celebrated my first real employment. We thought that our poverty and its unrelenting oppressive grief, seemingly endless at times, had finally come to an end. Mother cooked and served a complete supper of vegetables, yogurt, dessert, and our favorite beverage, buttermilk.

I took the whole family to an Indian movie, except Mother who did not want to go. It was a first experience for Darshan and Mamoon Jan. It was a romantic comedy. We arrived at the Rialto cinema hall after the movie had started. The theatre was almost full, and the only seats available were in the front row, much too close to the screen. From that close up, the pictures on the screen, including the people, were distorted and appeared like Pablo Picasso paintings. We laughed about it.

My Dream of Medical College

Within a few days, the results of the BSc examination were out. I had placed second in my class, missing the first position by just one mark, among some 30 students. I applied for admission to the highly reputed Glancy Medical College in Lahore, which was, until 1944, the only medical college awarding MBBS (bachelor in medicine and bachelor in surgery) and then MD. Admission depended on the aggregate marks obtained in three core subjects – botany or zoology, chemistry, and English – and the ethnicity of the candidate. The examination for a BSc degree was standardized throughout all the colleges (at least 30 in Punjab) that were affiliated to Punjab University.

Each ethnic group had a specific number of seats for admission, and their number was determined by that group's relative proportion of the total population in Punjab. Five places were allotted to Sikh applicants. The student's BSc score was the only criterion for admission. I ranked fourth from the top in the Province and was, therefore, selected. However, I faced two very difficult obstacles. First, how could I come up with the 364 rupees required to pay my admission and tuition fees up front for the entire scholastic year? Second, and by far the most challenging, how could I raise the money to cover four years of medical studies?

In retrospect, I wondered why I had not foreseen these problems. Probably, it was because I remained disconnected from reality and failed to see the limitations of the education system. My fragile dream was broken by a rude awakening when every avenue to find money was blocked off. It was a horrible setback that denied me the most important opportunity of my life. Outwardly, I kept a positive attitude, but inwardly, I was bitterly disappointed. When I look back on this period, I think of it as a personal failure.

The Bata Shoe Company

My job as enquiry officer required that I go door to door to verify that the number of household members corresponded with the number in their application for wheat and sugar rations, which were fixed on a per capita basis. I knew that the department had been created to tide over a temporary shortage of wheat and sugar. Given that Punjab's agricultural land was renowned as the biggest source of wheat and sugar cane, I knew that the shortage wouldn't last long. Since my job had neither a future nor a challenge, I was soon on the lookout for a better opportunity. Two attempts at securing overseas scholarships to study engineering and rubber technology were unsuccessful.

The Bata Shoe Manufacturing Company had been expanding very rapidly. It started in Czechoslovakia and quickly increased to 39 factories in different parts of the world, three in India alone. I found out from the owner of a shoe shop that they were looking for trained personnel. The factory in Punjab was unique and named Batapur. It was on the Grand Trunk Road, about an hour's bus ride from Amritsar. There was a huge complex of houses and bungalows for employees, a soccer field, recreational facilities, and a small shopping center, all of which were enclosed by a five-foot wall. Music with inspiring lyrics was blasted daily over a large area for an hour before starting time and during the two-hour lunch break.

In September 1944, one of my classmates and close friends, Bhagwant Singh Khaska, and I were hired by Bata. He later became a practicing lawyer and then Attorney General of Punjab. We were sent for training at the Calcutta Branch, Batanagar, which was close to a railway station named Nungi.

Batanagar was a well-planned city around a large factory on the banks of the Hoogly River, which is the mouth of the Ganges before it empties into the Bay of Bengal. There were residential quarters for workers, houses for management, bungalows mostly for European executives, a shopping center, restaurants, sports grounds, and two separate recreation clubs, one for Europeans who rarely mixed with Indians and the other for Indian employees. Bhagwant and I were given accommodation in the European quarters. These were also enclosed by a wall, and the entrance gate was guarded 24 hours a day by a sentry in uniform; all of the Europeans came from Czechoslovakia. During the following five months, we worked a five and a half day work week, 12 to 16 hours a day, during which we learned the art of making running shoes, labor administration, and management of personnel on the assembly line.

After our training, I was appointed foreman of one of the several assembly lines making running shoes at Batapur. A foreman's efficiency was measured by the quality and quantity of shoes produced by the workers on his assembly line. Efficiency, in turn, depended on a foreman's ability to motivate his workers, reduce absenteeism, and fairness in granting merit increases. I developed a good rapport with my workers and was soon acknowledged as a superior foreman.

Even though I was working, I continued to help my father in times of need. In March, he asked for my assistance with a transfer to Amritsar. After pulling some strings, I got him a temporary position at the Lahore Division Clinic. Meanwhile, Dalip Singh, the Superintendent at Lahore, was stalling the transfer. I'm sure this was because he wanted to make some financial gains, since he had a reputation for being imaginative and ingenious when it came to making money. In spite of this flaw, Dalip was a delightful person.

After waiting a while, I went to see Dalip. When I mentioned Father's name, his face lit up as if he had been expecting me. In the conversation that followed, I asked him to post Father to a clinic in Tarsikka, close to our home village. He then gave me upfront his wish list: two bottles of Johnny Walker and two pairs of Bata shoes. As for the shoes, he said, he was giving me a good deal because he knew that being a Bata employee I could get them free. I thanked him for being so thoughtful! I saw no point in contradicting him on the company policy, which to my knowledge had never given anything free to anyone.

The next evening, I brought him the scotch and the shoes, which I had bought from a retail store in Lahore. He thanked me and said that, for the moment, he would send Father to Attari, a town with a decent clinic halfway between Amritsar and Lahore. After a year, he would transfer him to Tarsikka. He kept his promise. Many years later, he was appointed professor of surgery at the Veterinary College in Hissar, where we eventually became colleagues.

Chapter 8: Tragedy Strikes

A Brother, a Friend, is Lost

Soon after his BSc examination at the end of April, Makhan accepted a job as a chemist at the Batapur factory and started living with me. His company brought me much joy, and our financial condition seemed to be improving, which made the whole family happy. We hired someone on a part-time basis to keep the house clean and cook our meals. Every Saturday, we would take the bus to Amritsar, visit our family, do our laundry, and press our clothes. Monday, we would catch the early morning train for Jallo Railway Station.

Once we went to Lahore to buy some cloth to be tailored at Batapur. I bought enough to make a jacket and a pair of pants for myself, while Makhan bought only enough for pants. On seeing his teary eyes, I asked him what was wrong. He wouldn't answer me. When I insisted, he finally replied that he, too, would like to buy some cloth for a jacket, but he didn't have enough money. I immediately paid for the cloth he wanted, which made him very happy. He was extremely sensitive and intense, but rarely expressed his feelings.

When he was 15 years old, Bibi had sent him with a ten-rupee bill to buy groceries. He asked me to go with him. On our way, we came upon a trickster by the roadside. The trickster had three inverted wooden cups (like wine cups) and a small red woolen ball. He would yell at passersby, "Double your money!" which caught Makhan's attention. We started to watch and saw that, with rapid hand movements, the trickster would lift the cups one at a time and move the ball from cup to cup or fake a move. Afterwards, he would ask a spectator to point out the cup hiding the ball. He would give a few trial runs in which his movements would be very slow so that spotting the cup with the ball was easy. This would raise the confidence level of the spectators, who would be lulled into betting. The trickster might even let such a spectator win a couple of times. All this time, Makhan had been watching, and then, all of a sudden, he wagered and lost all our grocery money. I was dumbfounded by his impulsive act. Of course, Bibi was very angry. We didn't eat well for a while.

Makhan had few shortcomings and many extraordinary qualities. He was sincere, dependable, a man of action with good manners and dry wit. We always worked as a team. When he was happy, his face would light up with a pleasant smile, and he would lightly scratch his short black beard. He was tall and graceful with dark brown hair. He had light brown, clear eyes, dimpled cheeks, prominent cheek bones, a fair complexion, and a sharp chiseled nose. Makhan had been named by my maternal grandmother because his fair complexion and handsome face reminded her of *makhan*, a smooth ball of butter.

In the middle of June, Makhan went to Amritsar by himself to find out the results of his examinations at Khalsa College. Two days after he left, I felt uneasy, an omen of impending catastrophe. This feeling followed me everywhere and wouldn't go away. That weekend, I left the factory at about five o'clock and took the bus to Amritsar.

When I opened the door, Darshan ran into my arms, weeping and wailing. She sobbed that Father had taken Makhan to the General Hospital because he had swallowed some opium, intending to commit suicide. She added that Makhan had found out that he had failed his examination. (In fact, he had failed in only one subject.) After getting the news, he had walked downtown to a licensed Hall Bazaar store to buy opium. Opium was available over the counter, since the government only regulated the price, quality, and purchaser's age. He had swallowed the lump of opium and walked the two and a half miles back home. When Father saw him stagger in, drowsy and in a state of confusion, he had rushed him to the hospital.

I hurried to the hospital. Bibi, Father, Surat, and Mamoon Jan were sitting around Makhan's bed. He was comatose and hooked up to a stomach pump to flush out the opium. Makhan was being attended by an internist whose antidotal measures were far from effective. His condition progressively deteriorated, and at about two o'clock, his respiration stopped, his heart arrested, and revival by every method failed. His body was wheeled out for an autopsy, and we were told to return at 10 o'clock the next day.

The loss was sudden and highly traumatic for everyone in the family. I, personally, had been deprived of an extraordinary brother, a loving friend, a soul mate. Together, we had walked hundreds of miles, worked as a team, played soccer, and lived a life, which I thought held some promise. Sadly, he probably thought that there was no hope and gave up. To Makhan, life had not been worth living, and he had seen no end to the difficult struggle.

Father, Surat, Mamoon Jan, and I returned the next morning with a cot to carry Makhan's body. His cranium had been cut open, his brain taken out for chemical analysis. The incision from forehead to the back of the skull had been coarsely sutured by someone, who was probably just as inexperienced in his trade as the internist who, the evening before, had tried to detoxify him; neither appeared to have much professional skill. Makhan's life could have been saved had the surgeon operated and removed the opium lump from the stomach.

His death was brutal and had a gruesome impact on our family. The four of us carried the cot with Makhan's body covered with white sheets. The road to the temple-morgue-crematorium complex, which was then outside the Hall Bazaar gate, was short but heavily traveled. Soon we were joined by many sympathizers who took turns shouldering the cot and chanting a refrain, "*Ram nam sat hai. Gopal nam Gat hai*" (In God's name lies the truth and salvation), thus sharing in our sorrow and grief. This sharing of grief by strangers is typical in India, especially among the poor. It is a hallmark of Indian society.

The temple priest very kindly sold the firewood for cremation on credit, since we did not have enough money on us. We were to pay him back when we returned to collect the ashes. We placed Makhan's body on the wood pile and covered it with wood all around. Father, wailing and crying, set the wood on fire, which was soon engulfed by flames.

The following three weeks was a period of terrible grief and mourning, shared by our uncles and other relatives who came to visit us. *Guru Granth* was read in its entirety as we prayed and meditated for the solace and comfort we so desperately yearned for.

A week after the cremation, our whole family went to collect Makhan's remains, which we placed in an urn. We had to leave the urn at the temple since we didn't have the money to pay for the firewood and service. Father and I were the only working family members, and the dismal salaries we earned only provided our family a precarious existence. There was hardly enough money to buy food. We were never able to go back and claim Makhan's remains. This left a deep wound in my heart that has never healed. I can only cherish the memories.

Chapter 9: In Search of a Job

Adventures in Bombay

Before the Second World War, Bata imported rubber from countries in and around the Indian Ocean. When these countries were occupied by the Japanese, India's rubber supply was cut off. Batapur then began using reclaimed rubber, processing old car tires with heat and chemical treatment. The stench generated by this process permeated the air in and around Batapur and was far more noxious than that of the waste disposal sites.

The Bata Company, like other manufacturing companies, polluted with impunity. At that time, there were no environmental guidelines, and if there were any, they were not enforced. Residents were unaware of the health effects of the stench and didn't care as long as they had jobs. For quite some time, I had been feeling lethargic, tired, and sleepy all the time. I would go home after work, collapse on the bed, and sleep until the next morning. I would eat in a stupor when woken up. I noticed, however, that this sleepiness and lethargy disappeared every time I left Bata. I knew then that I had to try to find another job. Unfortunately for me, unemployment was at an all-time high because industries producing war-related materials were closing.

Against Father's wishes, I decided to try my luck in Bombay. I had heard from friends that Bombay held immense opportunities. Once I reached there, I changed my appearance: I stopped wearing my turban, had my hair cut for the first time, shaved off my beard, and began hunting for an acting role in the movies, or "Bollywood," as it is now called. I met a contractor who supplied the film industry with extras. He took several photographs of me in different attire with my face creamed, adorned, and buffed with paints and powders, and my hair primped. This was an expensive introduction for a neophyte. It did not take me long to discover that the film industry operated on a network of connections. Landing even a minor role in films could take a very long time, and the wait was expensive. The idea of an acting future evaporated quickly.

In Bombay's suburbs, there was a place called Jogeshwari with a railway station of the same name. It had a rubber factory that manufactured running shoes and latex condoms. The factory bought ready-to-use reclaimed rubber and, hence, didn't have the pervasive stench of Batapur. The Japanese-owned factory had been expropriated at the beginning of the war by the Indian government who handed it over to a local Aggarwal family. The factory was famous for its labor strikes and hostile work force. Goons and hoodlums terrorized the feeble management. I accepted a job in the labor management section – a job which, to my dismay, later turned out to be as dangerous as that of a bouncer working for a nightclub in a lawless neighborhood.

The whole region surrounding Jogeshwari and its neighboring town of Andheri was rife with illegal activities. Two loosely organized gangs operated side-by-side, making every effort not to get in each other's way. A gang member was called *Dada* and his illegal activities *dadagire* (highhandedness). Both gangs ran lucrative gambling dens, probably in complicity with the police, trafficked in opium, and extorted monthly premiums from merchants as protection money. Those who refused to pay were harassed, beaten, and their shops burglarized. There was also widespread speculation on stock numerals. A gang accepted bets on any number from zero to nine and paid ten times the money staked on a winning numeral, which would be the last number of the closing price of cotton stock at the Bombay Stock Exchange. They may also have minted bogus coins. Gang members had their own ethics and knew one another. A few worked in the Jogeshwari rubber factory.

Hardly three months into my job, a foreman brought a worker named Shariff Khan to me. I was to give him his walking papers – that is a letter of dismissal and wages to date. According to management rules, I had no choice in the matter. As his final papers were being prepared, he started making abusive remarks, swearing at me, and hurling insults. He wouldn't leave, even after I handed him his wages and letter of dismissal. I tried to stay calm, but this made him even bolder. He declared that he would not leave until I went outside with him where he would show me who was boss. By that time, his rage had pushed me beyond my tolerance limit, and I decided to take the wind out of his sails. I grabbed him by the shirt and pushed him out the door. Surprisingly, he put up no defense or resistance and went away. Mistakenly, I thought that the matter was all over.

After about a week, I received a visit from a stranger named P. Singh. He introduced himself as the leader of one of the gangs. He said that Shariff Khan was his contemporary. I was surprised when he congratulated me on my courage and asked if I would be interested in joining his gang. After he left my office, giving me time to make up my mind, I felt overwhelmingly uncomfortable. Suddenly, security was my main concern. Being on factory premises, both my residence and the cafeteria were under constant surveillance. I decided it wise to restrict my outdoor activities to these two places, thus becoming a voluntary prisoner.

In the next few months, labor disputes at the factory kept sprouting. Longstanding basic issues of low wages, job security, and the absence of a coherent procedure to address workers' complaints remained unresolved. The owner decided to overhaul management and asked me and two of my colleagues to resign. I did and immediately moved to Santa Cruz, another suburban area of Bombay. I stored my suitcase and bedding with a family I hardly knew and, for the next month, slept on a deserted roadside, bathed in the adjacent ocean, and marched from factory to factory in search of a new job.

I took part-time employment, again in a shoe factory that was closer to central Bombay, where I recruited and trained workers in assembly line skills for manufacturing running shoes. I found my work satisfying, since teaching new skills to the jobless was acknowledged with thanks, which was a lot more pleasant than issuing pink slips. I worked from 8 am to 1 pm, which left me all afternoon to wander around Bombay's seaport. There, I would search for rich foreigners, sailors, or other visitors who wanted a tour guide. I avoided young enthusiasts with city maps, guidebooks, and tote bags, since they, invariably, preferred youth hostels or similar cheap places to stay and a bus to get there. They also usually wanted to sip cheap tea in roadside *dhabas* (eating places) and hunt for bargains. Within a few weeks, I instinctively learned to spot travelers who had come for pleasure and exotic cuisine, those who were anxious to check out historical sites and landmarks, take in a horse race, or buy something authentic. I would eagerly take them sightseeing and, better yet, help them buy souvenirs, jewelry, carpets, and antiques from shops that paid me a commission on their sales. Often, under the impression that I was giving them my "valuable" time free of charge, they would pick up the tab for my drinks and meals, thanking me profusely.

In a rare shopping spree, I bought two tight fitting shirts, two pairs of slim trousers, socks, and black leather shoes of a quality consistent with the sophisticated clientele of my new trade. I also started looking for a better postal address and eventually located a space on the second floor of a five-story hotel near my new job. The room had three large windows overlooking a shopping area and was a true model of open concept. It measured 35' x 25' and had 16 storage-cum-sleeping spaces along the wall, leaving a narrow passage in the middle. Each space was about 10' by 4' and had suitcases leaning against the wall with head space for pillows and mattresses. Everybody had their own bedding, which required frequent laundering to remove the reddish brown stains left by the bed bugs. We had no cooking or laundry facilities, but we did have a large restroom with four screened off toilets and four taps for showers.

When the factory opened in the morning, foremen from various sections would check for absentees and let me know how many workers they would need and what task each was to perform. I would then proceed to the factory's main gate where prospective workers waited to be hired. I would pick either those with prior experience or inexperienced ones whom I would then train during the morning hours. One day, I hired a young man, Uttam Singh, who had completed a two year diploma in leather shoe making. He had experience in many aspects of the leather and shoe trade. I took him to the general manager who hired him on the spot as foreman of a section that prepared leather components for the assembly line.

Uttam had grown up in Punjab where his father was a guard for the North Western Railway. On retirement, he bought land and built a house in Issapur, a village in the valley of the River Ganges. Uttam had left home a few months earlier in search of a better life and had drifted to Bombay where the only job he could find was looking after two cows that belonged to a *seth* (rich man). In return, he had been given meals and sheltered with the cows. He told me that he could no longer stand being struck by the cows' swishing tails, their tufty ends wet with urine. Since Uttam spoke Hindi impeccably – evidence of his good education in central India – I always conversed with him in Hindi. We spoke English with our European bosses who, out of pride or prejudice, had made no effort to learn any of the three local languages: Hindi, Gujrati, or Marathi.

Uttam quite happily moved away from the company of cows to a neighboring floor space. Since we were about the same age and had similar interests, we became good friends, spending most of our leisure time together. One day, Uttam was demonstrating to a worker how to cut leather soles from tanned hides using a metal die. The die was pressed down with an iron crushing board which he operated with a hydraulic foot switch. His right index finger got caught between the die and the crushing board. He underwent a lengthy operation to remove several small pieces of bone, but when his finger healed, it shriveled and lost all articulation. He was paid Rs490 from the Workers Compensation Board. A stockbroker who lived with us enticed Uttam into buying stocks with his windfall. Uttam couldn't make a spectacular run at the stock market to catch the wild price swing in time, as he had expected. Alas, the stock market plummeted, and so did Uttam's fortune.

Civil Unrest and an Independent India

From March 1946 on, the British Government had been actively negotiating India's independence with the Indian Congress and the Muslim League. As an outcome of these talks, Congress formed an interim government on September 2 of that year with Jawaharlal Nehru as Vice President. Congress' commitment was to elect an Indian constituent assembly and create a separate constitution for the ethnic minorities in various provinces. The interim government, however, was boycotted by the Muslim League, which wanted to secure the demands of the Muslim population before the British relinquished power in India. Consequently, interracial clashes resulted in the deaths of some 7,000 persons, the majority of whom were Muslims. As soon as the government was sworn in, a curfew was imposed in Bombay due to the riots. Uttam and I lived in an area that was sandwiched between ethnically opposed inhabitants. We waited for about two weeks and, seeing no sign of abatement, packed up and headed home.

I reached Tarsikka at the beginning of October. The village is about two miles from Kot Khera and about the same distance from my parent's land. The land needed a dependable method of irrigation, and Father had begun construction of a well, which was very tedious and time consuming. First, a circular brick wall had to be erected, starting from a solid foundation laid at the bottom of a pit dug to water level and rising to about 16 feet above the surface. The wall then had to be sunk deep under water by excavating within and below the foundation with a large heavy metal bucket attached to a chain. Underwater divers would then repeatedly dig down in the earth with the bucket which was pulled out by a pair of oxen. The dirt pulled out would be used to fill the hollow around the wall.

As the pit was dug and bricks delivered, Father realized that the work involved was much more than he had foreseen. Also, he started having differences with his deputy superintendent. The project had come to a halt before I got home. Bibi, whose inner strength would be energized by such crucial circumstances, asked me to help. I could never have refused. We got two of my cousins to come over. Surat, who had been studying at the Veterinary College in Lahore, came for a few days. We hired two divers, borrowed bullocks every day from different relatives in Kot, and built a shelter and temporary kitchen to feed everyone. By the beginning of December, we had completed construction of the well. Ironically, it is still waiting to be used even to this day.

In mid-December of that year, Rajinder, my children, and I had to attend the funeral of Rajinder's cousin at 118/10R. On the way, we stopped for a day with Rajinder's nephew who lived and studied at Jahania Mandi. He told me that his school had been without a science teacher for a long time and that Multan Division was in dire need of science and mathematics teachers. I went to see his headmaster, who directed me to Multan's District Inspector of Schools. I was hired on the spot and also offered a subsidy for the required nine months of study at the Training College in Lahore, which was due to start in January the following year.

The salary scale wasn't great, but the job was permanent, and there were fringe benefits – free tuition for my children up to university and the possibility of extra income from private tutoring. I did not have a particular inclination for teaching, but I was willing to make the necessary adjustments to embrace my new profession.

On the first of June, I brought my family to Tarsikka to spend the three months of summer break with my parents. Soon after, I received a letter from my headmaster, asking if I was interested in tutoring a small class of students. Lured by the additional income, I returned to Jahania Mandi before the month ended.

Chapter 10: Partition of India

The Role of Religion

Hinduism, a polytheistic and idolatrous faith had always been predominant in India. Several other religions, including Jainism and Buddhism, were also born on Indian soil and flourished side by side with Hinduism. All these religions had an important common feature – peaceful coexistence and avoidance of any form of violence. This strong, pacific element made a vast majority of Indians averse to warfare, which has been a distinct reason why India has been invaded and conquered so many times. Starting in 731, the Arabs extended their hold up to the southern border of Punjab, and in the 11th and 12th centuries, large waves of Muslim raiders from Turkey and Afghanistan sacked the prosperous cities of north India with utmost savagery, yelling for God and profit, but seeking only woman and plunder (Bristow, 1974). During their brief reign, they converted temples into mosques and Hindus to Islam by coercion and intimidation.

In 1526, Babur from Iran seized power violently and founded a Mogul dynasty, which ruled India for six generations in a father to son succession. Its emperors, Jhangir (1605-1627), Shah Jahan who built the famous Taj Mahal (1628-1657), and Aurangzeb (1658-1707), were puritanical orthodox Muslims who continued the persecution and conversion of Hindus to Islam and imposed the special poll tax, *Jizya*, on Hindus and their sacred places. The collective Hindu psyche never forgot nor forgave Muslims for the centuries-long subjugation and humiliation.

Mogul emperors, in pursuance of their religious intolerance, executed two Sikh Gurus, Arjan Dev in 1606 and Teg Bahadur in 1675. Bahadur's execution led the tenth and last Guru, Gobind Rai, to organize Sikhs into *Khalsa* (or pure), a militant brotherhood and warfaring political power to defy the Mogul empire.

Sikhs could now be readily recognized by their beard and turban. They had their own Punjabi script, *Gurmukhi* or Gurus' tongue modified from the Sharada alphabet (derived from Sanskrit). The pacific element of orthodox Indian religions – non-violence – had no particular appeal to Sikhs who adopted a militant attitude in defense of their religion. By 1767, the Sikhs had conquered northern India from Jamuna to Indus. In 1790, they began to unite under Ranjit Singh as their Maharajah, minted their own coins, and declared Sikhism as the state religion. Sikhs became unique by developing their own tradition, folklore, religious rites, and customs. They remained masters of Punjab until 1849 when they were defeated by the British.

During the British Raj, perhaps no other community in India prospered to the extent that the Sikhs did. They occupied key positions in the army, civil service, business, and industry. Six million Sikhs stood to lose the most from the creation of the new state of Pakistan. They reacted fiercely to the partition of India.

The 30 million Muslims of pre-partition India originated from Hindu ancestors or Muslim invaders. Muslims resembled Hindus in physical appearance, dress, and speech, but they had a distinct society and culture. They voiced concerns, however, about their identity and religious freedom. The Muslim League claimed to represent Muslim interests and demanded Pakistan as an independent Muslim state. The Indian National Congress, on the other hand, was a secular organization that represented India as a whole and claimed to be a potential successor to British rule.

During India's long struggle for independence, sharp differences in the political strategies of the Muslim League and of the Indian National Congress emerged. These differences arose from separate communal electorates for Muslims, Sikhs, Anglo-Indians, and Europeans. In 1917, for the first time, the British government created special religion-based constituencies and thus sowed the seed of communal discord by granting these political privileges. The British sided with the Muslims and Anglo-Indians. From then on, electoral candidates appealed to their own religious sects rather than to the public at large. The religious differences thus became worse and spilled over from politics to exacerbate inter-ethnic relations.

In August 1921, fanatic Muslims of Arab origin, *Moplahs,* rebelled and set up an independent *Khilafat* (opposition) kingdom in Malabar, South India. In their reign of terror, they converted thousands of Hindus to Islam and massacred many until the rebellion was suppressed in February 1922. Between 1922 and 1927, Hindu-Muslim riots took 450 lives and injured 5,000 people (Encyclopædia Britannica, 1962).

Mounting Uncertainty

In early 1947, political developments were shadowed by mounting public anxiety due to the uncertainty of the country's future. The population was being torn apart by its five major political parties. Hindu Maha Saba, including its activist limb, Bharatya Jan Sang, guided by fundamental Hindu doctrines, was a marginal political force. Slighted at not being invited to negotiate India's independence, it began to campaign angrily against carving Pakistan out of India. Their policies hardly inspired confidence that India's overwhelming Hindu majority would always remain fair to minorities. Akali Dal, another fundamentalist party, demanded an independent Sikh state in areas of Punjab where Sikhs were in the majority. Its leader, Master Tara Singh, who had been invited to the negotiations for independence, later dropped these demands in collusion with the Congress Party. The Congress, a secular and the most popular party, stood for a united India but did not have the confidence of the Muslim population. The Muslim League's members had been elected in many seats of the central and provincial assemblies and, therefore, represented most, but not all Muslims. The League remained uncompromising in its demands for an independent Pakistan and backed them with incendiary speeches and processions which, at times, went out of control.

On February 20, 1947, the British government announced its intention to hand over power to the Indian population. Only two political parties were to negotiate the terms of independence: the Indian Congress and the Muslim League. During negotiations, the Congress was willing to put the past aside and make generous offers to the League with political formulas to keep the country united. The Muslim League, in response, announced that August 16, 1946 would be a Direct Action day for Muslims to demonstrate their resolve to have their own state of Pakistan. Violent outbreaks occurred between Hindus and Muslims, in which Sikhs sided with the Hindus.

The rioting rapidly spread from Bengal to Bombay where I was then working. Forty-five thousand troops were brought in to restore order. A conservative estimate of those wounded or killed was 7,000, the majority of whom were Muslims. At the end of the Direct Action, Muhammed Ali Jinnah, the League's leader, declared, "What we have done today is the most historic act in our history ... This day we bid good-bye to constitutional methods ... Today we have also forged a pistol and are in a position to use it" (Farwell, 1989). It became clear to negotiators that partition of India was the only choice acceptable to the Muslim League. The Congress Party reluctantly agreed.

The British Parliament passed the Indian Independence Act on July 18, 1947. The line partitioning Pakistan from India was later drawn along the sub-district boundaries in the provinces of Punjab, Bengal, and Assam, grouping areas of Muslim majority into Pakistan. Thus, an independent state of Pakistan was born as a dominion of the British Commonwealth on August 14, 1947; that of India was declared a day later.

The logistics for a post-independent exodus – Hindus and Sikhs from Pakistan to India and Muslims from India to Pakistan – in terms of military support, transport mechanisms, compensation for properties left behind, and other contingencies were not well thought out beforehand. It had been clear all along that mass migration was inevitable, given the frequent inter-ethnic brutality and violence leading up to partition. The Declaration of Independence gave free reign to large-scale Hindu-Muslim riots with Sikhs siding again with Hindus.

The Hindus, Muslims, and Sikhs of Punjab were simple, courteous, and easygoing people, but they could become violent when incited by fanatical agitators. Law and order could swiftly turn into chaos. In Lahore, Pakistan, police made no effort to stop the Muslim mobs from burning a famous *gurdwara* and the 20 innocent Sikhs who had sought refuge inside (Bristow, 1974). In Amritsar, Sikhs in revenge stripped Muslims naked and hacked them to death. These incidents marked the beginning of a widespread explosion of frenzy and violent killing of innocent civilians on both sides of the newly created international border, letting loose the centuries-old religious-based hatred and prejudice. The police were unreliable, and human slaughter went on uncontrolled. On the eve of independence, waves of communal riots broke out on a national scale (Prakash, 1988). The Province of Punjab was divided and headed toward chaos and instability. And there I was living in the new state of Pakistan and my family with my parents in India.

A Home Becomes an Enemy Nation

I participated in Pakistan's flag hoisting ceremony at Jahania Mandi and, like other members of the minorities, accepted Pakistan as my new country with every intention of becoming a full-fledged citizen. Soon after, however, a large number of Muslim migrants started arriving from India telling tales of the horrors and atrocities that had forced them out of India. With every passing day, more and more Muslim refugees were arriving in cities and towns around Jahania, and as the pace of migration escalated, so too did the incendiary tales. Inter-ethnic relations were tense, giving rise to anger then to intense hatred with ever increasing momentum. Violence was about to erupt at anytime.

A friend who played soccer with me had inside information. He expressed concern about my safety and advised me to leave Pakistan within a week. At the same time, my neighbor, Sardool Singh, an overseer in the municipality, was also planning to leave. His brother, Jagjit Singh, a police constable in nearby Khanewal, was going to India with his constabulary and the Assistant Deputy Magistrate (ADM) of Khanewal by night train on August 26. The ADM was a member of the Imperial Civil Service with high-ranking powers similar to a session judge and county sheriff combined. Jagjit invited Sardool to leave Pakistan with him, and Sardool asked me to join them. We boarded the early morning train from Jahania to Khanewal where we would join the group headed for India.

At the railway station, local police were seizing luggage from travelers leaving Jahania; they made an exception in my case because some of the constables remembered me from a soccer competition (Police vs. the Rest of Jahania) held a few days before in which the Rest had won with me as captain and key player. They told me that the seized goods would be distributed among the refugees from India. We met with Jagjit in Khanewal where we spent the whole day. The city was overflowing with people bound for India.

Given the political turmoil, Jagjit thought that it would be safer if we traveled as policemen. He gave us extra uniforms, and that evening we met at the station with other members of our group: the ADM, his wife, his daughter and 15 policemen in uniform including the two "new recruits." All police personnel who had opted to move to India had been disarmed a few days before. As the train pulled up to the platform, we noticed a small coach occupied by a five-member military escort at the end of a long series of passenger wagons. Thinking that closeness meant better security, we took the nearest wagon to the coach. The overnight journey went without a hitch, leaving no harbinger as to what the morning would bring.

Massacre at Raiwind

The areas adjacent to the railway stations along the route were crowded with huts full of Muslim refugees from India who would surge to the platform unimpeded and rob passengers of their belongings. Members of the escort in our neighboring coach watched indifferently from their windows. At about 11 am, our jam-packed train reached Raiwind Junction, where almost all the passengers disembarked. We were all headed for Ferozepur, India, the next stop.

Raiwind railway station had a boundary fence and two raised platforms separated by a five foot high metal fence. The tracks for our Lahore-bound train, which had just arrived, ran along one platform, while the tracks for the Ferozepur-bound trains ran along a much wider main platform. On one side of this platform stood a long row of buildings and offices, including the stationmaster's office and the first and second class waiting rooms. The two platforms were connected by an overhead wooden bridge. When we got off the train, the ADM and the rest of the police staff went to find the stationmaster to ask when the Ferozepur train was due. Sardool and I stayed behind with the luggage, while the ADM's wife and daughter went to the first class waiting room.

By then, almost all the passengers had alighted and walked across the bridge and spread out along the length of the main platform. There were, however, still a few lingering on our platform. Sardool and I were sitting on the luggage, chatting with a couple who had entered our compartment at Chicha Watni, a station close to Montgomery. The man was the manager of the Punjab National Bank, and he told us in detail how he had carefully locked the bank's Rs11,000 in a safe before leaving. He was in the middle of a sentence when all of a sudden we heard a gunshot. The manager slumped to the ground, blood gushing from his neck. He had been silenced forever.

Sardool and I grabbed the manager's wife and took cover behind a large nearby tree. About 25 feet away, a soldier from our escort squad stood in the doorway of the coach, gun in hand, like a sentinel guarding against a possible assault. I could not take my eyes off him, and he and I quite often made eye contact. The first gunshot was immediately followed by the staccato of gunfire directed at the main platform where a large number of travelers had been waiting. The shots were coming from the escort coach. For five to ten minutes, ear-deafening sounds mingled with the victims' screams and wails. Meanwhile, the solitary gunman chose his victims one by one. Deliberately taking aim, he would pull the trigger slowly and watch them die.

Sardool, the manager's wife, and I watched in horror as the train started to move, carrying with it the firing squad. The main platform, which was now visible, was covered with infants and children, men and women, who lay dead or dying. It was a horrible image of death and human destruction. The inhumanity of the bloody scene was too much for me to bear. I was overcome by a chilling grief and paralyzing fear. I cannot begin to accurately estimate the number of people who were on the platform. I could be wrong, but counting roughly 70 passengers in each of about 30 wagons would leave 2,100 dead and wounded – a very real tally of the dimension of this cold-blooded pogrom. I shuddered at the ruthlessness of those who had killed mercilessly and with such violence.

A long period of silence followed the train's departure. Nothing moved. It was as if the world had come to an end. In utter despair, I took off alone and ran the 200 yards from the station to the village of Raiwind. I entered the first *haveli* with an open gate looking for shelter. I was fairly certain that its residents were Sikhs. A young man sprang up from his chair and told me to leave immediately. He said that the new inhabitants were from India and would not hesitate to kill me when they returned from their mission. I ran back to the platform and joined the ADM and the police personnel. All were safe and waiting. Apparently, they had not been able to locate the stationmaster; the buildings were all locked up and deserted. Eventually, they had found an army captain who was filling in for the stationmaster. He herded everyone into his office and bolted the door. Perhaps he knew what was going to happen. He had no information on trains which, according to him, were running without any schedule. Out of concern for our safety, he offered us the use of the first class waiting room.

As we were getting ready to walk over to the waiting room, a small train arrived at the main platform. It had three wagons carrying eight police officers in impeccable khaki uniforms and about 40 red-shirt coolies (red caps). The officers were armed with high-powered rifles. One of them came over and ordered us at gunpoint to march into a line on the main platform. Meanwhile, we watched in horror as the coolies loaded bodies onto the carriages, making no distinction between the dead and the dying.

Our little group stood facing the policemen. A tall man with beady eyes, bushy moustache, and shoulder stripes indicative of high authority stepped forward and addressed us in Punjabi. I thought, *This is the end. We are all going to die.*

The man fired off a lengthy speech, attempting to justify the savagery, claiming that it was normal retaliation for what was happening in India. He said he felt a sort of camaraderie with us since we were colleagues with the same professional ethics. He then added the strange rationale that we should work for inter-ethnic peace if we somehow made it to India. Finally, he told us that, while he could easily kill us on the spot, he was going to spare our lives. I breathed a sigh of relief. The policemen and coolies boarded the train with their grim cargo.

Soon, other survivors, who had luckily found shelter, began emerging, and by the time we bolted for the waiting room, there were 42 of us. We spent the night in constant fear of attack. Fear of dying was ever present as we sat there in a state of shock and confusion, our sense of reasoning and thinking paralyzed.

At about 10 o'clock the next morning, our train finally arrived with six fully armed Gurkha soldiers. The soldiers patrolled the platform while we boarded. Sardool, Jagjit, the bank manager's widow, and I got into the same wagon, parting company with the others in our group. The train moved slowly.

As it passed a big canal, hardly two miles from Raiwind, it was flagged down by a small group of people wanting to board. Sardool, who was closest to the door, helped one of them in. The man told us how his group of 31 people had dodged bullets by hiding behind the railway buildings. They had then fled to nearby fields where they had been greeted by a mob armed with spears, axes, and swords shouting some kind of a war cry. Many had been butchered. He had been chased by two men with swords. When his pursuers caught up to him, first he dropped loose coins, then paper money, and finally, his empty wallet. They had stopped to pick up the bait every time before resuming the chase. He made it to a canal and jumped in, swimming downstream while his pursuers followed along the canal bank for about a quarter of a mile before giving up the chase. When they were out of sight, he got out of the water and crept through the tall crops where he spent the night. Before daybreak, he resumed walking toward the railway tracks. When I heard his account, it dawned on me who the new residents of Raiwind were and what their mission had been.

Only 73 people had been lucky enough to escape alive from the ill-fated train. The events of the day had been so well timed that I doubted that they were coincidental. First, the arrival of the military squad precisely when armed mobsters barred the passage of fleeing passengers, and then the arrival of the coolies' train to dispose of the dead and dying. I wondered how many times this deadly enactment had been played out on India-bound passengers of the morning train at Raiwind station.

We reached Ferozepur, and from there we traveled by freight train to Jallundhar where we said goodbye to each other. I took a train to Beas and then walked for two days until I reached Tarsikka on August 31, circumventing Muslim villages along the way. I was never so happy as when I saw our house. Everybody ran out to greet me, and we hugged and cried. They were all immensely relieved to see me back home safe and sound. The horror of the massacre has stayed with me all my life. I still have nightmares.

The non-Muslim inhabitants of Tarsikka and Kot Khera were living under constant threat of a large-scale raid by Muslims, who made up about one-third of the population of Tarsikka. They and the people of the neighboring villages of Sangraun, Rasulpur, and Malowal had long been active sympathizers of the Muslim League and were well organized. August 1947 was tumultuous and marked by anarchy and mass murders, the likes of which Punjab had never seen. Father sheltered all my family at the Veterinary Hospital in Tarsikka, which was isolated and, therefore, extremely vulnerable. After about two weeks of imminent threats and fearing for our safety, we moved to the *haveli* in Kot Khera, thinking we would be relatively safe with our uncles and their families. Kot was in a state of constant alert. Six volunteers, armed with lances and swords, rode around the village in an all-night vigil while the rest of the men, awake and armed, waited for the alarm.

Uncle Isher cleaned up and polished the leather casings of his lance and sword and attached them to his saddle. He gave me a lesson on how to outwit the enemy in a battle for life and death. The vigilantes, whom he headed, were putting their lives at risk to safeguard families and friends. In mid-September, a small military contingent arrived and began escorting the neighboring Muslims to nearby holding camps and, subsequently, to Pakistan. It is now thought that, by the time law and order had been reestablished and the country was at peace, 6.6 million Muslims crossed the border from India to Pakistan, and 5.5 million Hindus and Sikhs from Pakistan to India. It is less certain how many people perished. The figure estimated by the army headquarters in East Punjab was one million (Bristow, 1975).

Peace Restored

During British rule, more than half of India's land was divided into some 656 states under the reign of Indian princes who were known as Maharajahs, Nawabs, or Nizams. They had gained possession of their states as a reward for helping the British conquer India. Their powers were defined by the British government. They took the state revenues as their personal income. Each state had a British Resident to make sure that the prince and his subjects remained loyal to the British crown. The rest of India was under the direct rule of His Majesty administered by the Secretary of State of India located in England and the Viceroy with supreme authority posted in India, both British citizens. British-India was divided into eight major provinces in addition to six commissionaries, or administrative regions. Each province in turn had several commissionaries which were divided into a number of districts comprised of perhaps 100 villages and towns with a total population of half a million people. Provinces were managed by a governor, commissionaries by a chief commissioner, and districts by a district collector (or deputy commissioner). A viceroy's immediate circle consisted of secretaries of different Indian departments, such as foreign affairs, law and order, tariff and customs, railways, income tax, civil and criminal law, etc. All the secretaries, governors, chief commissioners, and district collectors belonged to the Indian civil service, a small corps of about 1,000 highly qualified men recruited by strict competition (Cross, 1968). They controlled all government activities and provided a functional and stable government during the British period. The British administrative system again proved highly effective in reestablishing a rule of law in the turbulent post-independent India. The Indian civil service was then renamed the Indian Administrative Service and recruited only Indian citizens through competitions.

In India, the British Empire's hierarchical organization was guided by vested interests, but it did promote the well being of the population. The domination by a small group of foreigners over a much larger population of natives may be questioned on moral grounds. I believe that Britain's good intentions were never in doubt and their interest in India continued after independence, welcoming the country as a member of the Commonwealth.

Chapter 11: My Village

Kot Khera, Then and Now

India's partition fractured my village, and it never recovered. About a month after partition, a few army personnel arrived in our village and announced that all Muslims should assemble within two to three hours. They were then escorted to a nearby concentration camp. Our family witnessed heartbreaking scenes of parting. Relationships formed over innumerable generations had suddenly come to an end. Soon after they left, their houses, crumbled by the rain, were reduced to ruin and gradually disappeared, leaving only mounds of earth and empty spaces. And, at the end of the 20th century, there was hardly any evidence that they ever lived there. Their memories, too, would be forgotten.

In the 1930s, Kot Khera was full of people, life, and activity. But, at the new millennium, there were few inhabitants, many ruins, and not much vitality. The village is in a rich agricultural area with many exotic shade trees probably introduced by my ancestors. These include the banyan and the pipal (which belong to the genus *ficus* and attain formidable heights), the symbal (*Barringtonia asiatica L.)* that gives brush-like blooms with pink and white stamens, the white mulberry (*Morus alba)* which came originally from China and was brought for silk worms, and the tamarind. The only tree native to the area is the 20-40 foot high Acacia known for its dark bark used in tanning and its red heartwood for making lumber. It has beautiful fragrant flowers in bright yellow balls and conspicuous white spines.

In my youth, the village population was a mosaic of different trades, lifestyles, and faiths – Islam, Hinduism, and Sikhism. There was a *gurdwara* and a mosque, but no Hindu temple. Besides farmers, there were weavers, carpenters, blacksmiths and goldsmiths, a shoemaker, a barber, a professional jester, many merchants, two potters, and of course, the highly needed moneylenders. After 1893, when the descendants of the blacksmiths sold their lands, farming was exclusively the domain of the Khera families. Fifty-seven Khera families were listed then, and their numbers increased to an overwhelming majority in 1930. The remaining trades were conducted by other ethnic groups. All these occupations were handed down from father to son.

Apart from minor feuds, farmers enjoyed sincere and friendly relations with all artisans irrespective of their religion. The artisans were all poor, some more, others less, but the two groups were highly dependent on each other. Religious-based political parties such as Akali Dal or the Muslim League, were viewed with scepticism and failed to find a foothold in the community.

Next to farmers, the largest group by far were the Untouchable Sikhs (*Mujhbi* Sikhs). They were society's outcasts, and their social interactions were restricted to their own group. They lived in a segregated part of the village. Ironically, Untouchables in Punjab had long ago embraced Sikhism, a religion that preaches equality and condemns discrimination among its faithful. But nothing changed other than "Hindu Untouchables" became "Sikh Untouchables." In 1949, the Indian constitution declared any discrimination against Untouchables illegal, yet Indian society did not appear in any hurry to integrate them in its mainstream. In our village, Untouchable Sikhs had no particular trade. They did odd jobs for daily wages or worked as hired hands on farmlands on a yearly contract. Some were quite often blamed and, at times, prosecuted for theft.

There was only one Hindu Untouchable family; they skinned animals, tanned hides, and made country-style shoes for working in the rough fields. The head of the family along with his wife and son all worked, but they could not keep up with the demands of village farmers.

Weavers made up the third largest group in the village. They bought their homespun yarn from farming families who had made it from home-grown and home-winnowed cotton. They weaved this yarn into *khaddar*, a coarse fabric, which they sold either at a market in Amritsar, lugging it 18 miles on their bicycles, or locally to farmers' wives who made it into family clothing, stitching every piece by hand with needle and thread.

There were four or five blacksmiths who were in great demand and, consequently, became quite prosperous. They made, repaired, or sharpened ploughshares, sickles, saws, hoes, axes, spades, weeding blades, and choppers. Two carpenter families provided diverse services such as cutting trees, sawing lumber, making beds, doors, windows, ploughs, and wooden handles for agricultural tools. They also built walls and roofs and had ox-driven grinding machines to turn wheat into flour.

Cotton and wheat could be bartered for cough and cold remedies, salt, sugar, tea leaves, spices, lentils, and other grocery items at four of the village's retail shops. Their owners, Hindus or Brahmins, lent money and jewellery, at a high interest rate, to farmers who were eager to mortgage their land in return for a pretentious display of wealth at weddings or other special occasions. From one of these families came Maila Ram Kalia, a contemporary of my father and a famous lawyer who practiced civil law in Amritsar.

Of the two goldsmith families, only one was in the business of making jewellery. The other lived in a brick house, apparently well-to-do. The youngest member of this family was in the army. I would see him when he came to visit while on leave, riding horseback, and for the most part, loitering in the streets with coin-filled side pockets which he would jingle to attract my attention.

There were two Muslim potters who made earthenware pots and pans. However, earthenware was then in the process of being replaced by unbreakable tin-plated brass utensils. The potters got the message and switched to the transportation of goods, for which they acquired an assortment of donkeys, mules, and ponies for their new trade.

Our village had only one barber, a Sikh who belonged to the *Nayi* caste, literally meaning "nail cutter." He trimmed nails, cut hair, and styled beards, but his main occupation was to help parents find eligible bachelors for their daughters and determine their suitability by gathering information on their land, livestock, sub caste, and reputation in their village. This was important, since a marriage between inhabitants of the same village was prohibited. The *Nayi* and his wife were the negotiating link in wedding plans. They knew the cultural taboos that had to be strictly obeyed before, during, and after the wedding. He or his wife, or both, would escort the bride from her parents to her in-laws and back immediately after the wedding ceremony and in the subsequent two to three trips. Their fees for each of the many services from pre-wedding to post-wedding were fixed and came to a tidy sum. Business, however, declined rapidly when many procedural taboos were discarded, and parents began dealing directly with each other.

In those days, the goodness of a woman was equated with obedience – obedience to her father and mother-in-law, and to her husband, no matter how abusive. She was expected to work from dawn to dusk in silence and submission and bear male children. Daughters had no legal right to inherit their parents' property. There was an ancient practice, especially in poor families of northern India, to kill girl babies for many reasons, but particularly because parents could not afford a dowry. By the 1920s, the practice had all but disappeared. Still, parents considered a daughter as belonging to some unknown man, and their biggest preoccupation was finding a match in order to marry her off early. The raising and giving of a daughter in marriage was called *kanyan dan*, a "charitable act."

The *Marasi*, a tiny segment of the Muslim population in northern India, were known for telling jokes, singing, and playing music. Some of their jokes live on in folk memory half a century after they left for Pakistan. The *Marasi* were always asked to perform at weddings. These special occasions in a small village like ours were few, and so unless the *Marasi* was famous over a vast region, continuing the family profession was nothing short of a recipe for starvation. The single *Marasi* family in our village made a living helping farmers pick cotton and hoe corn fields. They also wove baskets with covers and pan-like receptacles or *shujj* from wild reeds. A *shujj* was a broad shallow container with a flat bottom, a high edge at the back and sides, and open in front. In the spring, we would see the Marasi shake the *shujj* full of wheat/chaff in a steady side to side movement with an occasional flip that helped retain the heavier grain at the back while moving the lighter husk gradually forward and out. The wind separated the two constituents according to their density. The flow of the chaff/wheat mix had to be adjusted every day according to the ever-changing wind velocity, a remarkable skill which they had developed and perfected. They were paid on the basis of output or weight of the wheat.

Kot Khera was an ideal place. When anyone died, we shared the grief; when someone was married, we shared the happiness. Poverty united the community. It was its only benefit. Our village experienced a sudden shock in September 1947 when the Muslim population was evacuated. It was a cultural casualty associated with empty houses, deserted street, abandoned dogs, and pervasive gloom. We lost a good deal of our common heritage and social solidarity.

During the 1980s, farming became increasingly mechanized in our village as part of a new trend that swept the whole country. Signs of this progress were apparent as early as the 1070s. Tractors replaced oxen, and the less effective one-share wooden plough was set aside for the multi-furrowed metal plough. The spring-tooth was in, and the wooden rake was out. The fast electricity-driven tube-wells took the place of slow irrigation wells.

Threshing machines were everywhere, and no one threw the wheat/chaff in the wind. Expensive agricultural equipment was bought jointly by several farmers who would then share the cost and its use. Chemical fertilizers were spread over the land that had been undernourished and overcropped for years. New strains of wheat and maize, promising earlier maturity, better yields, and pest resistance, became available. There it was, the famous "green revolution."

The available agricultural technology seemed to have been fully exploited to stretch land yield to the maximum. Even then, the peasants' financial conditions continued to decline, as the land, their only destiny, shrivelled with each generation. They had no easy access to higher education or a career in industry and lived with fading dreams, threatened with poverty while the world around them was enjoying economic prosperity.

The peasants in my native village have kept up a brave face and deserve much admiration for their patience, benevolence, and law-abiding nature. They still have faith in the current political system, although it has failed to provide visionary leadership, new ideas, or meaningful reforms. The government's post-independence record is one of failure, unless keeping peasants alive and on the land could be counted as a success.

In the 1980s, people of the Punjab were thrown into an extremely tumultuous period of rioting, during which a terrorist movement dominated by Sikh youths demanded an independent Khalistan. The movement's objective, legitimacy, and strategy failed to convince the Hindus and a sizeable proportion of Sikhs. Politicians who opposed Khalistan were murdered, and large donations were extorted at gunpoint to keep the movement alive. Terror prevailed in rural areas. The Indian government used military force to suppress it. Its action plan was simple and effective, though legally and morally questionable. Sikh youths were searched for in large-scale manhunts. Unarmed innocent suspects like those who were perhaps not so innocent, were given the same treatment – instant execution, no trial. Combat was cited as the reason. Several such atrocities by the army on Sikh youths have been recorded (Tully and Jacob, 1985). Counterterrorism by the government eventually succeeded in bringing peace and security to the region where lawful means had failed. While this upheaval was going on, Hindus, the last of the minorities, moved out of Kot Khera, leaving only Sikhs and Untouchables.

When Claire and I visited Kot Khera in the winter of 1990, nothing much seemed to have changed since my childhood. It was the same watery buttermilk that was used to wash down the hard-to-swallow cornbread, and the mustard greens were still cooked to semi dryness on a mud firebox fuelled by cow dung cakes. The old ox cart overloaded with grain and straw still crawled in a dead slow pace on its solid wooden wheels while bicycles, the sole means of transportation in the village, carried as usual up to three adults. The dirt on the streets was perhaps deeper than what I remember and still turned into ankle-deep mud during the rain. Just as in my childhood, drinking water was hauled from wells or hand-operated pumps, the elementary school stopped at the fourth grade, and toilets were still anywhere in the privacy of tall field crops around the village. Well-to-do politicians who live in the city, travel by car, and dine in fancy restaurants could never understand these people and their problems.

By the end of 2000, more than 12 families of farmers had vacated their houses in the village because it was more convenient to live on the land where they worked. The new feeling of security and safety plus the Revenue Department's consolidation of a farmer's scattered land parcels in one place provided the necessary stimulus to move from the village to the land. A few of the Untouchables received free land in other parts of the country and also left.

As it stands today, Kot Khera's legacy says little about its economic progress and even less about the rich culture and diversity of its past. In the last 70 years, the religions, variety of cultures, and differences in lifestyles so characteristic of the past have evolved into a much-reduced spectrum of interest, activity, and ethnic mix. Political follies have caused a sort of ethnic cleansing of what once was a vital multicultural community.

Chapter 12: Post-Partition India

A Political Detainee

At the end of September 1947, I began the task of rebuilding my life together with the thousands of others who had fled Pakistan. I traveled to Issapur to visit my friend, Uttam. His mother, the only one home when I arrived, told me that he had a very good job with the Deccan Shoe Factory in Hyderabad City. She gave me his address, saying that perhaps he could find me a job, too. At Mathura railway station, while waiting to go home, I ran into three young men who were on their way to Bombay where they had minor jobs in film studios. They offered to help me find a job there, so I decided to go with them. In Bombay, I ended up staying in a refugee camp that was set up in an empty army barracks at a place called Chambur. We had plenty of food, thanks to a charity organized by local Congress members. But I couldn't find work. Then, at the end of October, I received a letter from Uttam asking me to come to Hyderabad where I could easily get a job in his factory. I took the train the next day.

Hyderabad State covered about 82,000 square miles and, thus, most of the Deccan plateau. Its well-irrigated fertile land was the source of the State's revenue, with cotton, oilseeds, and hides (raw and tanned) its main exports. Hyderabad was completely surrounded by Indian Territory, and its ruler, Nizam Osman Ali, had refused to accede to India. Osman had heard the voices of the State's 86 percent Hindu population, but paid no heed to their demands for an elected assembly. On the contrary, he sponsored a private army of Razakars, Majlis Ittehad Al-Muslimin, under Kazim Rizvy to maintain Muslim supremacy in the Deccan.

The Razakars' relentless and nefarious activities and threats of violence had kept the Hindu majority subdued and in a state of suspense and fear. A large number of Hindu leaders who belonged to the Indian National Congress were detained without trial. News was censored by Nizam's government, which created a false impression that conditions in the State were secure and orderly. The authorities were determined to prevent, at all costs, a military takeover by the Indian Government. Uttam and I had both been taken in by this subterfuge.

By the time my train reached Hyderabad station, it was crowded with Muslim refugees fleeing India who thought that Hyderabad was a safe haven. I overheard refugees tell each other about the atrocities meted out by Hindus. This made me feel uneasy. I was already in Nizam's State, and it was too late to go back. The platform was full of noisy and disorderly Razakars armed with weapons that would have been obsolete even in the Middle Ages. Nonetheless, I felt intimidated, since my recent brush with death was still fresh in my memory. I did not dare leave the train and, instead, got down at Mahbubnagar, one of the next stations.

Once off the train, I asked how I could get to the nearest railway station in Indian Territory and where I could spend the night. Apparently, I had approached the wrong people. I was apprehended and subjected to an extensive police investigation that lasted more than two weeks. The police told me that Uttam had been tipped off and had left Hyderabad before they could question him. Absurdly, I was suspected of spying for the Indian government. This was because of the Nizam government's paranoia that the Indian army was planning an invasion. (It did occur, although much later in 1948.) There was no incriminating evidence to indict me, hence I was placed in detention and transferred to Hyderabad for further investigation, where I joined thousands of Congress workers.

From Hyderabad, I was sent to the Detention Center in Nizamabad, which was located in an old fort built long ago on a small hill outside the city limits. I was classified as a class B political prisoner. The Center held 550 political detainees. Safety had become a serious issue after a large Razakar incursion forced its way into the Center one night in March and beat up many of the detainees with steel pipes. I narrowly escaped injury. The detainees protested, going on a hunger strike and demanding an inquiry on the complicity between the Detention Center's supervisory staff and the local Razakar organization. The hunger strike was called off as soon as an inquiry commission was set up. All the detainees unanimously elected me spokesman, which I accepted with great reluctance. I met with members of the Commission and described the circumstances under which the safety of the Center had been jeopardized. I also gave details of my own detention, which I insisted was unjustified.

Within a week, five months after being apprehended, the Hyderabad State police took me to the border and put me on a train to Nagpur, the capital city of Central Province in India. All this time, I had been treated with courtesy and decency, but my incarceration had, nevertheless, caused me considerable emotional distress. My painful odyssey had brought me and my family five months of constant fear and worry.

Close to the main railway station in Nagpur, a refugee camp had been set up with about 30 huts made from palm trees and bamboo. The huts provided a shelter to families who came mostly from Sindh Province of former India. I was assigned a small hut which I shared with two bachelors named Krishan and Gokul. We were fed leftovers from the militia who were being trained across the road.

Krishan was in his early 20s and was subsequently enlisted in the police to be trained as a constable. Gokul was an expert archer who, even when blindfolded, could direct an arrow to a sound emitted from a target behind him as far as 20 feet. He left a couple of months later, joining a circus that happened to stop by Nagpur. Eventually, I was hired by the regional meteorological office as an assistant meteorologist on a three-month term job. The only work available after that was with the Nagpur High Court translating ancient revenue documents on land dispute settlements from Persian to English. It was a long-term contract with paltry pay. I turned it down.

I found out through the counselor at the refugee camp that the government was giving one-time subsidies to start up a small business. Given my experience in the shoe making industry, I came up with the idea of opening my own shoe business. I applied for and was granted a Rs2,500 subsidy. Uttam joined me and contributed Rs1,000 of his parents' savings. We both moved to Kanpur, where shoemaking was a cottage industry.

Under the trade name *Weara*, we bought ready-made men's shoes, which we then sold at a reasonable profit from our outlet as well as to retailers. Very quickly, we realized that our cash flow was insufficient for the required profit. To increase it, we needed to inject more funds in buying stock. I was at the end of my resources. Realizing that this business was not going anywhere and perhaps even heading to insolvency, I sold my share to one of Uttam's friends for Rs1,700, losing one-third of my investment. In the first week of December, I returned home to Beas, a small town between Jallundhar and Amritsar where Father was now posted.

University Once More

Before independence, the Province of Punjab had only one university which was located in Lahore. After independence, West Punjab and its capital, Lahore, became part of Pakistan, and East Punjab and its capital, Chandigarh, remained in India. Since both Punjab University and the Veterinary College were in Lahore, East Punjab created a new university soon after partition. It was also named Punjab University for the sake of continuity.

A new veterinary college was also opened in Hissar, first to accommodate students stranded from the Lahore College and then expanded, in December 1948, to teach a four-year course toward a BVSc, the degree offered by its affiliate, the new Punjab University. Since December was an unusual time for admission, an exception was made for the first class. Students would complete the initial two-year curriculum in one-and-a-half, which reduced the total length of study from four to three-and-a-half years and the number of annual examinations from four to three.

Father had obtained information on the new compressed courses through a government circular a few days before I arrived in Beas. Having failed in his quest to find me a niche in life, he urged me to take advantage of this opportunity, possibly thinking that education was the only alternative left. As always, Father had a lot of ideas, but none that would work without money. Paying for Surat's education (now in his third year at the new college), he said, had stretched his income to the limit. If I decided to go to college, I would have to fend for myself. Father was, however, willing to look after my young family until I graduated.

I knew full well that my financial resources were inadequate; nevertheless, I entered veterinary college after New Year's Day in 1949, hoping against hope of winning a scholarship. As it turned out, my money ran out after one year. Soon after, though, I did get a scholarship from the Punjab government worth Rs70 a month. Still, there was a shortfall of Rs20 a month. I pleaded with Father to help me make up the difference. Not only did he agree, but Mother and Rajinder also decided to help me by selling some of their jewelry. I will be forever grateful to them for helping me out.

Teachers at the College acted as co-examiners at the annual qualifying examinations. This gave them considerable authority over the students. All of them, and that included professors and demonstrators, were very helpful except one, the professor of histology and physiology. This professor taught Surat and me during the first year and a half. His was an unorthodox and austere method of teaching that discouraged students from asking questions or initiating a discussion. Surat had difficulties with him and, as a consequence, failed in one of his subjects. Surat warned me that if this professor found out that I was his brother, I might be his next target. I wanted an easier ride, and so we decided to keep our relationship secret. Our deception lasted until after the second year's examinations.

Classes were held at three different locations: the breeding farm, the veterinary clinic, and on the college campus. I needed a bicycle to get from one place to the other ,and so I decided to go to the *haveli* and retrieve my old one from my Khalsa College days. It had no mud guards and no brakes, although some vestiges of the old brake system clung to the tired frame as a testimonial to its glorious past. I made frequent use of my feet to brake, and this was very hard on my shoes. To make a sudden stop, I had to jump off and pull the bike back with all my might. It was a spectacular gymnastic maneuver that I acquired through trial and error. My friend and roommate, Rajinder Bhalla, thought it was very funny.

My bike was a notch above those of my classmates. Everyone knew who it belonged to and, because it didn't have a stand, I could lay it down anywhere without fear of it ever being stolen. When I left Hissar, I offered it to Mr. Joneja, the architect of its many repairs. He deliberated for two days before accepting the offer, saying that given all the time he had spent on it, it now had sentimental value for him. I knew he was getting emotional when he took it from me.

Veterinary studies gave me a sense of purpose, but throughout, my education remained more of an involvement than a commitment, a pursuit rather than devotion for which I had much enthusiasm if not dedication. In all three annual examinations, I stood first in my class in aggregate marks and in all but one subject. In the final year of my BVSc, I received the highest marks since the degree was first introduced.

A Job as Veterinarian

East Punjab and PEPSU (Province of East Punjab States Union) provinces had a similar hierarchy which rose from the Director of the Veterinary Department to the Secretary of Agriculture and then to the elected Minister of Agriculture. The director and the secretary had sweeping discretionary powers which they used indiscriminately and, quite often, capriciously. A director in complicity with the secretary had complete control over veterinary assistant surgeons (VAS) with respect to promotions, granting study leaves (within India), or accepting resignations. He could easily refuse a VAS' resignation and could even prohibit him from applying for a job elsewhere. Thus, a director held a VAS hostage to the provincial veterinary department.

In 1950, the Indian Agricultural Research Institute began granting research fellowships in alternate years to veterinary graduates for advanced studies in pathology, bacteriology, parasitology, physiology, and genetics. The fellowships were highly contested with criteria for selection based mostly on academic achievements. Confident of winning one, I applied for a fellowship in pathology for the 1953 academic year. For the ten months until the fellowship actually began, I would need a job that wouldn't box me in. I asked the Director of the Punjab Veterinary Department for conditional leave without pay in the event that I was selected. He refused. However, the Director of PEPSU Veterinary Department agreed; I joined PEPSU's services and took charge of the clinic at Faridkote in the middle of July.

My Young Family

In the first nine and a half years of my marriage, I was either a student dependent on my parents or wandering from place to place in search of a job. I lived with my parents under appalling conditions in grinding poverty. Our rented house in Amritsar did not even provide adequate shelter from the rain or from the rats that burrowed in through the mud floor. We had very little to eat other than *chapattis* and watery soup to which Bibi would add a few grains of lentils or beans. During this entire time, Rajinder spent only two, maybe three months a year with me, for a total of about 21 months. She found our living conditions too harsh and chose to live with her mother, Chinty, who was financially well off. The two shared a deep bond and enjoyed each other's company. Rajinder's father had died soon after our wedding, and her two brothers, who were also well-to-do, came to live with them as a joint family. In a way, I was happy with the arrangement, since I saw no point in having her share my life of austerity and misery. I had no other choice. I had to get an education.

From the very start, our marriage was unusual. Rajinder and I never lived together as a normal married couple. We were strangers in a strange marriage. I was a stranger as a husband and as a father. I failed to imprint on my children as I should have. Nevertheless, their welfare remained of paramount concern to me.

Our first three children were born during this period. My first child, a girl named Surinder, was born in 1941. After reading the news in a letter from

Rajinder, Makhan and I immediately went to see her. She had a brown complexion and a very pretty face. I held her in my arms with great care and was filled with joy and love for her. Unfortunately, we could only stay for a couple of days, since we had to return to classes. Jagtar, my second child, was born in 1943, and my third, Balbir, in 1945. Again, I learned of their births through letters and saw them for the first time when Rajinder brought them on one of her brief visits.

In November 1946, while I was helping dig the well in Kot Khera, Rajinder, Surinder, Jag, and Balbir came to stay with me in a small, temporary hut. Rajinder helped Mother with the cooking, and we all slept on the floor, which was quite crowded. Once, in the middle of the night, a thunderstorm struck without warning. Heavy rain permeated the shelter's thatched roof, and we had to evacuate. Rajinder gathered our clothes, and we started walking to Tarsikka. Rajinder carried Balbir while I carried both Surinder and Jag. Surinder, who was then five years old, was so afraid of the thunder and lightning that she refused to walk a step. By the time we reached Tarsikka, we were all soaked and exhausted. This was the first time that we had experienced something together as a family.

After the well was dug, I took my family to Jahania Mandi where I had a job teaching mathematics and science. The next six months was the longest unbroken period I had spent with my young family. I enjoyed playing with the children and shared their joy. I tried to let them know that they, indeed, did have a father, even if he had been absent most of their lives.

The following year, I brought my family to spend three months of summer vacation with my parents at Tarsikka. I gave Father the money that I had saved. He was very pleased. Surat was also home for the summer. He loved to tease Jag who at four years old was very fond of going for walks in the fields surrounding our new well. Surat would invite Jag for a walk to the well three to four times, waiting a few minutes in between which he would introduce an irrelevant subject to change Jag's attention. After every invitation, Jag would walk up to his mother, hug her, and tell her that he was going for a walk in case she might miss him and wonder where her "chun" (moon) had gone. We all thoroughly enjoyed this, as we did so many other affectionate and intimate moments. Alas, our time together was brief, and I had to return to Jahania Mandi for tutoring. Partition and independence of India followed, and in its aftermath, the massacre at Raiwind.

Rajinder's mother, brothers, and many other relatives were still in

Pakistan where a large population of Sikh farmers inhabited hundreds of villages surrounding Jahania Mandi and all around Multan District. During this crisis, they all got together – an estimated 100,000 of them – and trekked a harrowing 220 miles across Pakistan, carrying their belonging in ox-wagons and on horseback. They walked in caravans several miles long with only a few sawed-off shotguns for defense. Along the way, they lost a few lives warding off hoodlums in isolated scuffles. They took short breaks to attend to childbirths, deaths, and cremations in the three-week journey to the border at Harikay Pattan and to safety. It was a story of human fortitude and compassion which, like many other heroic deeds of those times, was never fully told and was lost forever in the post-independent era of turmoil and destruction. Rajinder's mother and brothers lost their home and fortune. From that point on, Rajinder and the children would live with my parents.

In addition to death and destruction, the post-independence era ushered in a sinking economy and record-high unemployment. All my efforts to earn a decent income had come to naught. At the end of 1948, after selling my shoe business, I joined my family in Beas. I had not seen my wife and children for 18 months. Father and Bibi had been looking after them, and Father had become a substitute parent to my children while I was away. When I arrived, the children looked at me as they would a stranger. Rajinder received me with mixed feelings, happy and yet upset that I was failing to provide for the family. My parents welcomed me back and seemed to understand my difficulties. I wanted to be a father to my children, but first I had to get a job, which was extremely difficult to find, given my qualifications. I had faced so many rejections that I started to question whether I would ever be able to provide for my family. This, then, was the reason why I decided to pursue veterinary studies at Hissar.

As a student, my parents were again the guardians of my children. Father was gentle, patient, and loving with them, surprisingly more so than he had ever been with me. Bibi had a natural gift with children and provided a warm environment with her cheerful disposition. They both gave Rajinder and my children a secure home and opportunity for education, which I had so far been unable to do.

While under my parents' care in Tarsikka, Rajinder gave birth to Awtar on April 2, 1951 at about midnight. Intuitively, I was there a few hours after his birth. The following year in July, I was finally able to assemble my whole family to live with me in Faridkote. My fifth child was born in February

1953, a girl whom my mother-in-law named Paramjit (Jyoti) when she came to help us for a few days. Jyoti was the only child born in my presence. She had a lovely face, smiled all the time and resembled Awtar. I now had three daughters, and the worry of their future marriage and dowry started to gnaw at me.

The clinic in Faridkote was in the centre of fertile land owned by well-to-do farmers. I never charged for services at the clinic since fees from house calls provided me with an adequate income. For the first time in my life, I had an inkling of what it might be like to be rich; also, it was extremely gratifying to be appreciated. My veterinary practice had its own challenges and rewards, but it wasn't enough. I just didn't have what it takes to make a good practitioner. The job demanded action, physical strength, and above all, good relations with the public. It was as much business as science, and I wanted more science. I enjoyed solitude, which I would spend in thought and reflection. I needed to satisfy my curiosity with scientific investigation.

Rajinder and I invited my parents to spend a few days with us. We gave them presents and bought them good clothes. It was a delightful visit. The day before they arrived, I had done my first major surgery – castration of an expensive colt. It had gone well, and before actually doing the operation, I had read the surgical procedure at least three times. When I told Father about it, he jokingly replied that he had done so many of them that he could now do them with his eyes closed. I replied, "Not fully closed, but maybe half-closed?" Father nodded, and we both laughed.

Faridkote had a strong field hockey team, largely due to Sarup Singh who sold sporting goods. He had played for India in the International Tournament held a few years before in South Africa and was known for playing barefoot. (As a child, he had been too poor to buy running shoes, and later on, he had found them too uncomfortable.) In the fall, he entered our team in the All-India Dhyan Chand Tournament in Delhi organized to commemorate Mr. Chand, a wizard and strategist of the game. Mr. Chand had captained the team that won the first Olympic title for India in 1928. I feel privileged to have had the opportunity to meet and talk with Mr. Chand. We won three matches but lost in the quarter-final.

Postgraduate Fellowship at Mukteswar

The results of our fellowship application came in, and I was delighted to have been selected for a scholarship in pathology. Surat also won one in bacteriology, and we both left for Mukteswar in Uttar Pradesh to start our research for a master's degree at the Indian Veterinary Research Institute.

The Indian Veterinary Research Institute was founded as the "Imperial Bacteriological Laboratory" on December 19, 1889 (according to a foundation stone later discovered) in the city of Poona (now Pune) near Bombay. The laboratory was moved to Mukteswar sometime in 1892. Mukteswar was a secluded mountainous village in the Kumaon Region of the Himalayas with only a few houses, 7,500 feet above sea level. Mules and donkeys transported almost everything required to build and furnish the Institute, as well as the employees' houses. The laboratory equipment and breakables had to be carried on human backs over 60 miles of strenuous mountain paths from Kathgodam – the closest town accessible by train. The Institute was built at great monetary expense and human effort. Its research activities in the beginning were mainly geared to producing vaccine and sera for livestock which required using cows for research. The isolated location safeguarded the secrecy of its operations, especially from those who held the cow in reverence.

Surat and I traveled by train to Kathgodam, then journeyed the last 12 miles by bus and horseback, reaching Mukteswar on June 4, 1953 in the evening. Rajinder, Jag, Awtar, and Jyoti joined me a few days later, while Surinder and Balbir stayed behind, partly because the free accommodation provided by the Institute was not large enough for all of us.

The Institute had become a branch or part of a large complex built at Izatnagar in Barielly, the main Veterinary Research Institute for research in physiology, parasitology, and genetics and also for the production of dried vaccine. The Mukteswar branch became the Department of Pathology and Bacteriology, conducting research on microbial diseases, while the pathology section remained at Izatnagar. For several decades, the section had been providing diagnoses on pathological tissues sent by field veterinarians from all over India. As the flow of tissues dwindled, practically stopping by 1950, its mandate changed to conducting independent research. Two positions had been added, and Mr. P.R. Krishna Iyer, the Research Officer, was ordered to move to Mukteswar. Mr. Iyer, the only pathologist at the Institute, strongly resisted the move.

There was no evidence that the move, which was more for administrative expediency than in the best interest of research, would happen anytime soon. Mr. M.R. Dhanda, the head of the Pathology and Bacteriology Division at

Mukteswar, was not a pathologist but, by virtue of his position, was my titular teacher and was to assign me to a pathologist. With Mr. Iyer's refusal to move, Mr. Dhanda had no one to assign to me. However, he did provide me with some help and suggested the research project for my thesis – microscopic changes caused by Rinderpest virus in cattle and goats. The choice was determined primarily by the readily available tissues from animals routinely infected with the virus. He gave me laboratory space, an outdated rocking microtome to cut sections, and permission to buy stains and chemicals from the store. I could also borrow books and journals from the Institute's library. However, what I needed most and didn't get was a mentor, someone knowledgeable who could confirm my observations and validate my interpretations. Pathology, being a practical and not a theoretical science, requires developing the knowledge, sense, and skill to recognize what is or isn't an abnormal alteration when a tissue is examined with the naked eye or under a microscope.

After six months, I had acquired all the tissues needed for my thesis; some were preserved in formalin bottles, but most had been converted into microscopic slides. I put in a request to go and work with Mr. Iyer in his laboratory at Izatnagar. It was refused. However, a number of favorable events occurred. A relatively large laboratory fell vacant when its protozoan research was discontinued upon the retirement of Dr. H.N. Ray, who was a well-known protozoologist. The building became the new pathology section, and Mr. Sundaram was appointed its new research assistant on his return from prolonged treatment for tuberculosis.

The Izatnagar pathology section sent over about a thousand bottles containing tissues preserved in formalin, a collection dating back to 1912, along with their diagnostic records. I was given a new rotary microtome that could cut much better sections than the old rocking antique. With the help of Sundaram, I processed and cut thin sections for slides from all these tissues, except for a few that had become too hard. I stained them as warranted. Armed with these stained sections, a textbook on pathology by W.A.D. Anderson, and scientific journals, I became a self-taught pathologist.

Once my thesis was completed, Mr. Iyer looked at some of the slides and confirmed the important findings. I submitted my thesis at the end of 1954 to Punjab University in partial fulfillment of the requirements for my master's degree in veterinary science.

A Soccer Field in the Mountains

The Mukteswar Branch formed a veterinary colony that sprawled over a vast hilly area surrounded by stone huts, the homes of local inhabitants who had lived there for generations. Most of them were employed by the Institute as technicians, animal caretakers, and other such jobs. Many worked in shops, the local hospital, and the school. In the centre of the colony was a soccer field which, in marked contrast to the miles of sharp hills and narrow plateaus, sat on a level area.

Soccer was a significant activity in Mukteswar, which otherwise was a dull and dreary place. It did not have any entertainment other than two clubs which provided a limited social outlet. Therefore, many members of the community came to watch us practice and to socialize. Surat and I introduced a spark of interest for spectators when we turned practice play into match play by dividing players into rival teams, office vs. laboratory, or technical vs. support staff, etc. These matches soon became the highlight of life in Mukteswar.

This soccer field had been built or, more appropriately, excavated, thanks to Dr. J.T. Edwards who was the Director of the Institute long before the Izatnagar Branch came into existence. Apparently misled by the office superintendent, Dr. Edwards had not obtained prior sanction from the government to build the soccer field, believing that the expense, roughly Rs100,000, was within his authority. Dr. Edwards, himself a good player, encouraged everybody to play and coached a team for the Kumaon Hill Championship. Winning this championship was his dream, but it was never realized.

An audit of the Institute's expenses revealed the irregularity which led to a contentious interrogation. Following archaic colonial laws, Dr. Edwards was compelled to relinquish his duties on the spot and given notice to leave Mukteswar within 24 hours. The rushed decision raised many questions on the judiciousness and fairness of the verdict. According to local soccer players, the decision had tarnished management but not Dr. Edwards, whom they remembered with warm affection. To them, he was a fine gentleman with a fierce passion for soccer, and best of all, he had left behind a cherished landmark, for which he had paid dearly.

What most of the local people didn't know, however, was that Dr. Edwards was a towering scientist of extraordinary vision. He attenuated the Rinderpest virus by 50 or so serial passages in goats – a less susceptible host.

The resulting virus lost its virulence, but still retained the ability to confer life-long immunity to cattle. This virus provided the seed vaccine for mass vaccinations that eventually eradicated the highly contagious and rapidly fatal Rinderpest disease from India (Datta, 1954). Dr. Edwards lives on in the history of veterinary medicine as he does in the history of Mukteswar.

By 1953, we had organized ourselves into a viable team and easily won the 1953 Kumaon Championship, which was an annual event in Almora, a big town 14 miles from Mukteswar. We played again the next year and, in the final match, competed against the Almora Soccer Club. Our opponents had seven players who were on a short leave of absence from the Indian army. Our team found their strategy disheartening, if not outright frightening. As soon as one of the army players got hold of the ball, all their players would lunge forward yelling, "ATTACK! ATTACK!" like a war slogan. Their hysterics and furor gave the soccer field a semblance of a battleground.

Our team was limited in tough experience. We had never witnessed military exercises and were intimidated by these tactics. Our opponents scored a goal more out of sound and fury than by superiority of play. After about 15 minutes, they were threatening to score again, but their momentum and dominance lost most of its edge when one of their noisy and aggressive players collided in midair with Surat while heading the ball. He fell bleeding profusely at the eyebrow. The incident, the watershed of the match, was not serious but was enough to rattle their team.

The ball traveled briskly up and down the field. Both teams missed scoring opportunities, and the defense lines on each side were tenacious. Our team was having a hard time finding the right rhythm to get the ball through their goal posts. A few minutes before the final whistle, we charged their defense with flair. Their goalie jumped up in the air and impulsively punched the ball with full force. It struck my head, knocking me to the ground where I lay unconscious. When I regained consciousness, I realized that I was being carried by my teammates and thought I had been badly hurt. Then I heard them shout that my heading of the ball had scored a perfect goal. They had picked me up in a frenzy of joy, not realizing that I had passed out.

Play resumed, and the match eventually ended in a one all tie. The tournament committee decided to determine the winner by the toss of a coin since the army players had to leave that very evening to report for duty. Our team won the toss and the trophy for the second time in a row; albeit not as deservedly as the first time. The captain of the opposing team borrowed the shield from us. They all stood in a line, hugging, kissing, and touching, one by one, the shield with their foreheads in reverence – a most impressive gesture. The photograph of our winning team was still hanging in the hall adjoining the entrance of the Institute's main building when Claire and I visited the Institute in 1990.

Research at Mukteswar

In the 1930s and 1940s, the Pathology and Bacteriology Division had earned a stellar reputation in Middle Eastern and Far Eastern countries for its significant contributions to veterinary microbiology. The Division was well equipped, and there was no shortage of funds or facilities. Dr. Datta, the Director of the Institute, had impressed me with his research acumen. He had done most of the research for his DSc degree from a British university at our Institute. I entertained hopes that, maybe, I could get this coveted degree in the same way. I had my heart set on a research career, but there were two disconcerting issues that would affect my career aspirations.

The first was that a new researcher had to follow the customary progression through three non-laboratory positions prior to reaching the laboratory post. The lock-step advance to reach the laboratory took effect only when there was a vacancy in any of the laboratories; this could take years. The non-laboratory channel had been bypassed recently by the direct appointment of a research assistant upon completion of his nine months postgraduate training at Mukteswar. This precedence, I thought, might also work for me.

The second issue pertained to authorship of research papers published from the Institute. Normally, the Institute's administrative authority validated research conducted there as a formality, since the author alone is responsible for the accuracy of the published results. The authority cannot dictate who the authors are. It is understood that the senior author (in the case of multiple authors) has done most of the research, while a single author has done all of it. A scientist's published papers are a mobile billboard of his/her productivity. This work, along with the quality of research, is a scientist's claim to fame.

According to Indian tradition of recognizing research in those days, credit for published papers went to the hierarchy; as head of the Division, Mr. Dhanda felt justified in claiming to be the principal investigator for papers published by his Division. However, many wanted to redress the imbalance, saying that credit was being unfairly diverted from those who really did the research.

From 1955 to 1960, my guide, Mr. Dhanda, was cited as the senior author of 16, and the junior author of one out of the 17 papers published from his Division (Dhanda, 1955-1960). The duration of a project from research to publication is highly variable, but four to five years would be considered average. The above period corresponded with my two-year stay at Mukteswar. During all that time, I never once saw Mr. Dhanda work in a laboratory. These publications, however, portrayed him as an extremely busy scientist.

The hijacking of research findings by authorities was accepted at the Institute. There was an often repeated joke in the scientific community about a scientist who had sent a paper to his laboratory in-charge for validation. The in-charge added his name before the scientist's and forwarded it to the division head who also added his name ahead of the two already there. The paper was then passed on to the director of the institute. The director inserted his name ahead of the three already listed, struck off the last name, or the name of the scientist who had done all the work, and sent the paper out for publication. He thought that four authors were too many!

A Rocky Road to My Master's Degree

My master's thesis was approved early in 1955 by Mr. Dhanda and the other two examiners appointed by the university. In order to qualify for the degree, I had to obtain 50 percent qualifying marks in the remaining four examinations: theory and practical in my major which was pathology per se, bacteriology, virology, and immunology, and in my minor – veterinary medicine. (This second subject was quite broad and rather vague, somewhat of a rehash of all the subjects I had already passed in my BVSc.)

Following approval, I started preparing for the exams. The Bacteriology Laboratory in Mukteswar had a large stock of pathogenic bacteria and viruses, and its courteous laboratory staff helped me learn to isolate, culture, and identify important bacterial and viral agents. After two months there, I went to the Institute's Parasitology Laboratory for a month, where I found a large collection of disease-causing flukes, tapeworms, and roundworms preserved as specimens. By April, I was ready.

I had earlier applied for the post of research assistant in the pathology section where I was working. My bond with the PEPSU Government would not matter, since the Indian Veterinary Research Institute was endowed with overriding powers and could recruit qualified employees from any provincial government. The week before I was to leave to write my theory exams, I received an appointment order asking me to report immediately as clinician of experimental animals (research assistant of out kraals). I sought an interview with Mr. Dhanda and politely apologized for my inability to accept the offer, explaining that the recent precedence of direct appointment to the laboratory had prompted me to apply. I added that working anywhere other than in the pathology laboratory would be prejudicial to my career. He insisted that I join and refused even to see my viewpoint. From his attitude, I deduced that senior authorship of my research may have been on his mind. He took my rejection as an act of arrogance and an insult to his high office, even though I had been extremely conciliatory. At the end of the interview, it became clear that applying for the job had been impolitic and that the outcome of my impending exams was now in jeopardy.

I wrote my exams under a cloud of pessimism and started hunting for a job. I applied for the position of meat inspector in the New Delhi municipality, thinking that its round-the-clock slaughterhouse would provide me with a good source of material for continued research. Also, working at night would free up my days to pursue university studies. I didn't get the job, probably because the president of the municipality had guessed my hidden agenda. Meanwhile, the results of my examinations were posted, and my worst fears were realized. I had failed in the practical of my minor – veterinary science – and would have to retake all four exams. I had only one more chance to qualify for the degree.

In September 1955, I applied for work as a veterinary assistant surgeon in the PEPSU Veterinary Department, again at the initial salary of Rs100, and was posted to Patiala, the capital city of PEPSU. Not even a month into my job, Surat stopped by to see me on his way to England for a nine-month course of Diploma in Bacteriology. He absolutely had to have Rs300. With not a sou in my pocket, I borrowed the money. I had great difficulty paying it back.

The Pathology Section of the local Medical College provided diagnosis of biopsies to a large general hospital. The staff of the section was very kind and accepted me in their laboratory where I studied micro slides from biopsies for about two hours a day. My family came to join me in Patiala, except Surinder and Balbir, who remained with my parents. Bibi and Father showered them with so much attention that they chose to live with them in their early life.

Chapter 13: L'Institut Pasteur in Paris

A Dream Come True!

One afternoon in Patiala, a Scottish lady rushed into the Veterinary Clinic carrying a lap dog in her arms. The dog was comatose apparently from licking quick lime from the whitewashed walls of her house. In tears, Miss Sullivan pleaded with me to save her pet. I immediately injected adrenaline, and the dog regained consciousness. I gave it a second injection of emetic (a vomiting agent), and it then vomited the lime. Within five to ten minutes, the dog was up and running around, wagging its tail. It was a miraculous recovery, beyond my own expectations. Miss Sullivan grabbed me and showered me with hugs and kisses.

A spinster and senior to me by about 25 years, she taught English at a local school for children of aristocratic families. I knew that the school covered a broad curriculum that included languages, so I asked her whether there was anyone on staff who taught French and could help me learn it. She immediately volunteered her services, saying that she had studied French in school and knew it well enough to teach it. She invited me to supper and a first French lesson that very evening. Miss Sullivan did not invite Rajinder because the visit was a teaching session and not a social evening. Any doubt in Rajinder's mind about this meeting was quickly dispelled when I told her that Miss Sullivan was well past Bibi's age.

At supper, Miss Sullivan introduced me to a Miss Mueller, a friend and colleague who was about her age. Miss Mueller taught German and had come to India after World War II. She had studied French as a second language as an adolescent in her hometown in Germany and spoke very little English. Both ladies took it upon themselves to give me French lessons. Their teaching credentials included a visit to France, more precisely to Paris. Miss Sullivan went for a week on a sightseeing trip, and Miss Mueller was there for a month during the German occupation in the Second World War. They were the only foreigners on staff at the school and had few, if any, social relations with others. Feeling isolated in a strange culture, they welcomed me as a daily visitor and thoroughly enjoyed conversing with me.

Initially, I made some progress in learning and comprehension. Soon, though, my progress stalled. Their pronunciation and intonation differed from one another, probably influenced by their mother tongue. Initially, we conversed in fractured French, but gradually this changed to English, which was easier and more convenient. Eventually, the learning sessions transformed into social evenings.

My French lessons came to an end the first week of April 1956 when I was promoted to Lecturer and transferred to the newly created PEPSU Veterinary School in Faridkote. The school had been established in such haste that its annual expenses, including staff salaries, had not been budgeted for the new year. It took the provincial government five months to pass a retroactive supplementary budget for the school through the legislature. During this period, I lived on borrowed money. I ended up spending so little that I was able to save a small sum which I put aside for the future.

At the end of April, I wrote the exams for the MVSc degree and this time qualified. Soon after, I applied for a French government scholarship to study at one of my favorite research institutes, L'Institut Pasteur in Paris. I appeared along with 22 other candidates in a competition held at the French Embassy in New Delhi. I rated my performance as dismal, but a letter dated September 29 informed me that I had won one of these scholarships! It really took me by surprise. I eagerly began studying French on my own.

Rajinder was pregnant again, and Bibi invited her to stay with them in Ramdas for the delivery. Rajinder along with Jag, Awtar, and Jyoti left at the end of September. Our last child was born in the middle of October, a girl we named Nickky. Upon hearing the news, I immediately went to see her. She was a healthy and happy baby, but very small. During my visit, I told everyone about the French scholarship. They were all very happy for me. Once more, I had to ask my parents to care for my family while I went to France. They were reluctant at first, but eventually agreed. My sister Darshan had graduated from Punjab University with a Bachelor of Arts degree in 1955 and a Bachelor of Training in 1956. She qualified as a teacher and was appointed to the same middle school in Ramdas where my children were studying. She took them under her wing, and I credit her for my children's good work habits and love of education.

On my return, I applied to the Minister of Agriculture for a two-year leave of absence, which had been recommended by Mr. Pritam Singh Brar (Mr. Brar was Director of the Veterinary Department.) and, subsequently, by the elder of the well-known Randhawa twins who was the Secretary of

Agriculture in PEPSU. Approval by the Minister of Agriculture was all that was needed and was considered a mere formality. My application stayed in the Minister's office for three and a half months! I was ready to leave for Paris when he finally gave the sanction on condition that I sign a bond to serve the government for five years on my return, in whatever capacity the government might choose. I felt trapped. The timing was inopportune to fight back. I could not leave without signing, lest the government make it an issue with the French. I signed the bond under protest. (Soon afterwards, PEPSU merged with Punjab Province, and all its assets and liabilities, including me, were handed over to the Punjab Government, my future bond holder.)

The French Government scholarship included a monthly stipend in French currency equivalent to about 35 British pounds and a return ticket from Paris to Bombay on the French Liner Messagerie Maritime. With the money I had saved, I bought an air ticket from New Delhi to Paris, three travelers checks of five British pounds each and a railway ticket from Faridkot to Old Delhi. I was also able to buy a heavy, but attractive brown leather suitcase which has, since then, accompanied me on every important journey. I still have it and treasure it as a memento of my destiny.

I arrived in Old Delhi the day before my departure. I found a cheap hotel after some shopping around and haggling, which might have gone on longer had I not been tired out from walking with the suitcase heavily loaded with clothes and books. The next morning, I took a taxi to Connaught Place where a courtesy bus would take me to the airport. I had to use all my bargaining skills to get the taxi driver to stay within my budget. By the time I got on the courtesy bus, I only had two paisas left, which were worth about one penny. This was yet another occasion when poverty reached out to me. Nevertheless, I was thrilled about the prospect of traveling abroad. I looked forward to a lot of fun and excitement.

On November 8, 1956, an Air India flight took me to Bombay. That same evening, I boarded another Air India flight bound for Paris. The plane was supposed to make a fueling stop at Cairo, but was rerouted through Baghdad and Rome because of heavy fighting in the Suez Canal.

Our plane was small with a capacity of about 60 seats arranged in 15 rows on either side. The front two seats on the left were occupied by an elderly English couple with the husband in the aisle seat. I sat directly behind his wife, and the aisle seat on my side was not occupied. As soon as we were settled and the plane airborne, an announcement came that supper would be served in half an hour. The gentleman in front ordered champagne. The order immediately caught my attention, and the air hostess and gentleman became the subjects of special observation. The couple downed their drinks, and the hostess gathered the empty bottle and glasses. I noticed that no money had changed hands.

I had never tasted champagne before. The only alcoholic drink that I was familiar with was "firewater," a cheap Indian whisky with a wild kick to match. Even when generously diluted, it produced intense burning sensations as it traveled to the stomach. Drinking it was no different than drinking red chili sauce on the rocks. To me, champagne was a luxury that only maharajahs could afford. I got the impression that it was part of the meal. So, I ordered a bottle which was served to me right away. I felt content, sipping champagne and nibbling on peanuts.

My happy feelings soon evaporated when the hostess reemerged with a bill. I gestured with my hand for her to bring her head closer to mine and whispered in her ear, "How come you did not charge the gentleman in front of me?"

She replied, "He is entitled to it because he is traveling first class."

She then gave me a choice to pay in either British, French, or Indian currency citing the equivalent prices. I took out one of my three travelers checks but before I could sign it she told me that she could not accept it.

"You must have more money," she said.

I answered, "This is all I have."

She couldn't hide her surprise and asked, "What will you do in Paris with no money?"

I straightened my neck, proudly raised my head, and informed her that I was going to study for a doctoral degree on a French Government scholarship. I expressed my regrets for putting her in this predicament. Sensing my delicate economic condition, the good-natured stewardess wished me luck and left with a big smile.

After supper, I experienced a strong desire to have a cigarette, but didn't have the impudence to ask the stewardess for a pack of cigarettes. I decided to suppress the urge, at least for the moment. At about midnight, our plane landed at Baghdad. The passengers were asked to go for coffee in any one of the three airport waiting rooms. I entered the first one and sat at a large oblong table. I was followed by a smartly dressed gentleman who sat across the table from me. He opened a metal can containing Capstan cigarettes, which were then somewhat expensive, and sold in cans of 50 or packets of 20. He placed the can and a matchbox on the table after lighting up. It renewed my urge to smoke, but I was too shy to ask for one. I was running low on nicotine, experiencing withdrawal and extremely vulnerable. The sight and smell of smoke was taking its toll on me, initiating Pavlovian reflexes of salivation and a display of intermittent glances. Unwittingly, I would look at his face, at the smoke and the can, and then reverse the order.

He had a keen sense of observation and got the message. He spontaneously introduced himself (I have forgotten his name), saying that he was Secretary to the Maharajah of Patiala and was accompanying him to England on a special mission for the Indian government. He offered me a cigarette, which I accepted. He gave a quick push to the can and matchbox, and they came gliding down the table's slick surface. I took a cigarette from the can. He told me, "Take more." I took out two more. He then said, "No, no, take more!" and backed up his offer by turning his head sideways. Taking this as a sign of encouragement, I surreptitiously filled up my inner coat pocket with enough to last me at least another day. I sent the can sliding back to him with the same maneuver that he had used earlier. We reboarded the plane, and after a long stop in Rome and engine trouble that developed just before Paris, we landed safely at Orly airport.

I was in a buoyant mood. I exchanged one of my traveler's checks which gave me about 54 French francs, 50 in bills and four in coins. A shuttle service from Orly to the bus terminal in Paris cost me two francs. I exited the terminal and looked for a taxi. I had planned to spend the night in a hotel within walking distance of the Bureau du Comité d'Accueil pour les Boursiers du Gouvernement Français (Office of the Welcoming Committee for French Government Scholarship Holders). The office was on the Boulevard Raspail. Directly across the Boulevard was the well-known Institut de Langue Française which was a famous landmark. I tried to make the taxi driver understand in my Sullivan-Mueller French that I wanted to go to a hotel close to the language institute. He couldn't understand me. So, I produced a letter from the Committee which gave directions in French. After reading the letter, the driver nodded, and I heaved a sigh of relief.

We reached the hotel after a short drive. The driver asked me for the fare. I pulled out all the coins that I had, about two francs, and presented them to him on my outstretched hand. Since I was not familiar with the currency, I asked the driver, in my best French and then in English, to take what was the appropriate fare. He grabbed all the coins in one clean swoop watching me gleefully, and shaking his head up and down, he uttered loudly, "Merci! Merci! Merci encore!" and drove away.

I entered the hotel lobby with my leather suitcase. The concierge behind the front desk gave me a bill, and I paid the amount written on it. I asked him if there was a place to eat nearby, first in French and then in English. I was having great difficulty making myself understood in either language. He went on at length and at breathtaking pace with an accent unfamiliar to my ears. From the few words that I could decipher, it appeared to be French. Seeing that I was confused, he started all over again, this time with a different vocal sound, pitch, and accent, but at the same rapid firing pace. I asked him to explain again, slowly and in English. He bemusedly retorted, "What language do you think I was speaking?" He paused a moment, then he clapped his hands and burst into a hearty laugh saying, "Monsieur, your French is better than your English!" I laughed to keep his company knowing fully well that the joke was on me. Thus, on this humorous note, my journey from India had come to an end.

The magnificence, beauty, diversity, and eccentricities of Paris impressed me and gave me a singular joy that I had never experienced before. I was amazed at the network of underground metro service that connected the metropolis with its environs. It was, indeed, a marvelous engineering feat of subway stations and interconnecting tunnels. Almost any place in and around the city was within walking distance from a subway station. The trains followed each other like ocean waves with thousands of commuters riding to and from their workplace in minimum time for a nominal fare. The metro's efficiency had made all other modes of travel in Paris irrelevant.

There were uniquely designed majestic edifices arranged in straight lines for miles on end enclosing pedestrian sidewalks and wide boulevards and a median lined with trees all along. Walking there was delightful.

I knew that the Romans and Italians had graced their sculptures, sketches, and paintings liberally with the male figure. French art was infused with the lush contours of the female, as if to capture warmth and delicacy and please the esthetic senses. For the first time, I realized that this fascination with the female form had been transferred to the clothing industry. Indian clothes always tried to hide a woman's figure, burying her in multilayered garments that were designed with chastity in mind. No wonder a well-clothed Indian woman looked like some kind of diva or deity. Any effort to peel away a layer offended an Indian's sensibilities. Nothing of that sort could be seen in Paris. French fashion was more about physique, physiognomy, and silhouette and not just about cotton, silk, and chiffon. Clothes were fashioned imaginatively as if to stir up fetishistic fantasies. They were teasingly transparent, flirtingly brief, and seductively fitting. And then, there were those coffee-sipping onlookers watching girls go by, sitting in outdoor glass-walled terraces found all over the city serving café au lait and insomniac decoctions named Turkish coffee.

The romantic style of tailoring was matched by quirky necking and smooching of lovers glued to walls, corridors, and pillars. The scene of two lovers in a tight embrace with extremely busy lips and tongues seemed too banal to attract anybody's attention, but not mine, for I had never seen that before. I found it very unusual, since in India even holding hands was sure to raise eyebrows. I watched furtively in the beginning and found that this cultural oddity seemed to increase in intensity and frequency with the approaching dusk.

Within a few days, it became evident to me that Parisians were unique, courteous, witty, easygoing, and given to talking especially with their hands, arms, and shoulders. While sitting in a cafeteria eating my first lunch, a middle-aged man in construction clothes approached my table and pointing at my glass of water asked, "What are you doing with that?" I answered, "I plan to drink it." He then told me that water was only for washing clothes and hands which he emphasized by rubbing his hands together. He then erupted in laughter saying, "Si vous buvez de l'eau, Monsieur, vous aurez des grenouilles dans votre estomac!" (If you drink water, Sir, you will have frogs in your stomach!) He laughed and laughed and left me with a "Bon appétit!" and the thought that he might well have a point. This was my third encounter in two days with French humor. Although, I could not quite understand the wit in their punch lines, I found so much warmth in people everywhere, and that made me feel welcome.

A Guardian Angel

The Welcome Committee informed me that my application to work at the Pasteur Institute's Virus Laboratories had been rejected. As a consequence, the Committee had arranged for me to work with the Central Laboratory of Veterinary Research which was close to the Veterinary School at Maison-Alfort on the outskirts of Paris. The laboratory was not recognized by the

Université de Paris at Sorbonne for a doctoral degree, but I still had the prerogative to change to any laboratory that was willing to accept me.

I started looking and was turned down wherever I applied, probably because of my difficulties with French. Depressed but not dismayed, I ran into a highly respected professor-scientist in physiology, Mademoiselle Lebreton, who turned out to be my guardian angel. She read my credentials while listening to my litany of unsuccessful efforts. Suddenly, she looked up and asked what laboratory would be my first choice. I was at the point of saying any one would do, but replied "Le Service des Virus" at the Pasteur Institute. She immediately picked up the telephone and dialed its head Dr. Lépine. She told him, "C'est un garçon extrêmement intelligent...." I could only guess that Dr. Lépine had agreed, but there was a minor hitch. The Service was recognized by the Sorbonne, but Dr. Lépine lacked the accreditation as guide for the doctor's degree. This was readily resolved by Professor Lebreton, who became my official professor, with Dr. Lépine as my actual guide. Dr. Lépine wanted me to start on the coming Monday. (This happened on a Wednesday.) My angel immediately snapped back "Pourquoi pas demain?" (Why not tomorrow?) because otherwise he will only hang around in the streets of Paris for four days. I was at the Service des Virus at 8 am the next morning.

On my very first visit, Dr. Lépine spelled out the details of my research program, which was the normal schedule for all trainees. I had to work independently in all eight constituent research laboratories of the Service des Virus. These were: Poliomyelitis, Reckettsial, Cocksachi, Rabies, Foot and Mouth Disease, Electron Microscopy, Animal Colony (that performed special surgical procedures), and the Media Room (that made different media for growing cells in cultures from scratch).

My progress from one lab to the next depended on how quickly I acquired the necessary knowledge, technique, and skills. Individual supervisors would coordinate my moves between laboratories. By the time I reached the last laboratory, I should have decided on a research project for a doctoral thesis. I should also have the necessary information to convince Dr. Lépine of its feasibility and originality. If he was convinced, he would give me the go ahead. Whenever there were sufficiently interesting and original findings, I would have to discuss these with him and seek his approval. He would review the writings before sending the thesis on to Professor Lebreton who would then review it and present it to the Faculté des Sciences in Sorbonne. The duration of the research for the degree was not stipulated in terms of time; its length was determined primarily by a candidate's efforts, ability, and results.

Dr. Lépine, a tall and graceful man known for not wasting time or mincing words, was one of the best virologists of his day. He helped shape my future, offering me limitless learning opportunities. For the first time in my life, I felt in control of my own destiny.

During my sojourn in Paris, I lived in Cité Universitaire. It was founded in 1922 and occupied a large area along the Boulevard Jourdan in the southern part of Paris. It accommodated about 4,000 students in some 22 maisons (hostels) built by different countries, each providing its own maintenance. India did not have a hostel, so I chose to live in the Maison des États-Unis which was built in 1928. In addition to housing facilities, there were tennis courts, soccer fields, a swimming pool, two large restaurants, a theatre, and a medical center. The whole area was picturesque; there were numerous flower beds and tree-lined streets. Food for the students was subsidized by the French Government.

The Cité's population came from all over the world and formed a community in which I blended right away. Each hostel hosted monthly "soirées," inviting students from the other hostels for social evenings. I took an active part in discussions on issues that were intended to bridge the diversity between students.

I studied French until November 15, 1957 at the Alliance Française. That first year, my daily routine from Monday to Saturday, was to wake up at 4:30 am, study for three hours, work at the Institute from 8:30 am to 6 pm, walk to the Alliance, eat in its cafeteria, and attend French classes from 7 to 9 pm. I would be in bed before 10. Other than a few hours off on Sundays for sightseeing, there wasn't much entertainment, and soccer was certainly out of the question. This wasn't how I wanted to spend my days in Paris, but I had to get my degree as soon as I could.

There were a few social graces at my workplace that were as interesting as they were endearing. Shaking hands every morning on arrival was ritualistic. Once when I forgot, one of my fellow workers, his face etched with concern, enquired about my health. In addition to the handshake, ladies were expected to receive a few gentle words about their looks, clothes, or perfumes. One could go as far as "Vous êtes ravissante, madame"(or mademoiselle) (You are ravishing or delightful) without getting into trouble or being labeled a flatterer.

We also had food provided by professional caterers that was served in our cafeteria. Quite often, a few of my colleagues' spouses who worked in neighboring laboratories joined them for lunch. Every time they came, they would kiss and whisper in confidence two or three amorous phrases. Two that I heard quite often were "Mon choux," "Mon lapin," (my cabbage, my rabbit). The symbolism of the rabbit to cuddliness was clear to me, but I could not figure out how the cabbage fitted in.

In September, ten months after I started, I had completed the circle around the virus laboratories. I then spent two weeks studying the commercial production of Foot and Mouth Disease vaccine at L'Institut des Fièvres Aphtheuses in Lyon. While there, I also visited its veterinary school that claimed to be the first in the world. I was taken on a tour to another institute (Marois) near Lyon that manufactured commercial sera and vaccines for veterinary use. Its owner spent half a day showing his laboratories and hosting a delicious lunch. He asked me to sign his visitors' book that had a separate page for each country displaying the country's flag. For India, I was the second to sign after Dr. G.L. Datta who was the Director of the Veterinary Research Institute when I worked for my Master's degree. The owner asked if I knew him.

By February 1958, I had completed my research on the Foot and Mouth Disease virus, and by the end of March, my thesis and summary were with Paris University. The University's method for thesis evaluation was unique. The thesis summary was sent to other universities and select institutes in France. There was a 40-day waiting period during which the candidate first had to settle adverse comments if any had been received (which was bad news). Thankfully, none came in my case, and so the university fixed a date to assess my thesis and selected two examiners in addition to my official advisor. Open discussions were held, in which the public – generally academia and researchers – was encouraged to participate.

The examination of my thesis began with the presentation of an abridged version lasting 45 minutes, all in French (the university's language). This was followed by comments and questions by the examiners and then by anyone in the audience. At the end, the examiners deliberated in confidence on the originality, significance of results, validity of the findings, and general quality of answers, arguments, and counterarguments. They would determine whether my thesis met the standards required for a doctoral degree and, if so, with what "mention" (recommendation).

Everything went smoothly. I qualified for Docteur-ès-Sciences degree with mention "très honorable" of the Université de Paris on May 17, 1958. Dr Lépine, in his certificate dated May 29, 1958, stated:

"Mr. Khera proved to have excellent intelligence, scientific interest and professional conscience... I personally congratulate Dr. Khera for the research accomplished in my service and under my guidance and issue him the present certificate as a testimonial, for those acquainted with him, of the high esteem in which I hold the person and research of Mr. Khera."

I had realized my dream of obtaining a doctorate from the University at Sorbonne, which was perhaps the oldest university in Europe, dating back to the first decade of the 12th century. Its Faculty of Science was founded in 1666. The university served as model for Oxford, Cambridge, and many other North European universities (Robertson, 1989).

I took pride that L'Institut Pasteur framed so much of my life. It was founded by Louis Pasteur in 1887 and was built with public donations. It was an institute that received no public funding for its operations and was run by the commercial sale of its biological products. The Institute stood for certain unchanging values. It did not exist for itself; it existed for the sake of people who, in turn, revered it as a symbol of learning.

On my first visit to Gare Montparnasse, a railway station near the Institute, I picked up a small piglet for my research. I had to wait in a long line for cargo delivery. When I reached the counter, the clerk who was tickled pink with my squealing goods asked what it was for. When I told him, he instructed me to come straight to the counter next time because the Pasteur Institute had a priority claim to railway service.

I found that all French people I had the privilege of working with were irresistibly charming. They presented themselves as ordinary people; however, to me, they were very special because of their affection and warmth. I made many friends in the Virus Laboratory and received countless invitations to meet the families of Dr. Lépine and senior staff members. On these occasions, I thoroughly enjoyed French culinary pleasures, especially the wines.

When I left the Institute, I mentioned to Dr. Lépine that I had felt rootless when I first arrived in Paris. But when I left, I felt a part of the family. I owed so much to the generosity of the Institute and its workers. He responded that he would never reject anyone from India whom I recommended.

Chapter 14: Return to India with High Hopes

Life with a Doctorate

In order to refresh my knowledge of pathology, I spent a month at the Pasteur Institute studying a collection of microscopic slides that had been prepared from diseased tissues by the pathology laboratory. After that, I took the Messagerie Maritime at Marseilles on June 17, and we docked in Bombay 11 days later. Its familiar surroundings immediately brought back memories of the times I had chased wealthy tourists to make a living. Two days later, I was home at Ramdas. My family had been counting the days, anxiously waiting my return. Everybody was extremely happy to see me, proud that I had completed my education. There were celebrations and festivities and lots of food. Father had retired six months earlier and moved the family from the rent-free residence at the clinic to a rented house. Everyone anticipated that I would get a good job, and we would all live happily ever after.

During my absence, Father had betrothed and married Surat to Surinder Mahli, a girl from the village of Sialka, about ten kilometers from our village. She happened to be the daughter of Mohan Singh Mahli, the Director of Veterinary Services in Punjab. I borrowed some money from Darshan (she thought I was a better loan risk now) and reported for duty to Mr. M.S. Mahli. He wrote to the Office of the Secretary of Agriculture proposing my appointment as assistant disease investigation officer.

Since my student days, the Veterinary College had gone through two important changes. First, the position of assistant disease investigation officer was transferred from the Veterinary Department to the college. Its new job description included the diagnosis and control of infectious diseases in sheep and goats. The other was a change in the mandate of the college. It was to be modernized into a research institution of higher learning in veterinary science.

The Honorable Pratap Singh Kairon, the Chief Minister of Punjab, had hired Mr. P.N. Nanda to oversee implementing this challenging new mandate. Mr. Nanda came from a rich and well-connected family. He studied in England where he obtained his MRCVS (Member of the Royal College of Veterinary Surgeons) diploma. He started as superintendent, PVS I, with the Punjab Veterinary Department and, in short order, became the Animal

Husbandry Commissioner of India, the highest government position a veterinarian could aspire to. When Mr. Nanda retired, the Hon. Kairon hired him immediately, probably impressed by his meteoric rise and title "Rai Bahadur" (brave noble) conferred by the British Government for loyalty and distinguished service. He was given a five-year contract at an undisclosed high salary. The upper hierarchy thought he was well suited to manage the changing role of the college and created an aura around him. And, too, he was tall and handsome.

The Veterinary College had two vacancies: assistant disease investigation officer in PVS II and professor of genetics in PVS I. All PVS appointments (class II starting salary Rs250 and class I Rs350) were made by the Secretary of Agriculture directly or, if he chose, by selection through competition held by the Public Service Commission. Appointments could be challenged, whereas those made by the Commission were not. In either case, appointments had to be approved by the elected Minister of Agriculture, which was a mere formality. The Minister never wanted to meddle in the Secretary's affairs unless the legitimacy of an appointment was questioned. The Secretary's position at that time was vacant, but the Assistant Secretary was filling in.

After seeing Mr. Mahli, I spent ten days with Surat who was working at the Indian Veterinary Research Institute in Izatnagar. After an appropriate period of time, I sought an interview with the Assistant Secretary in Chandigarh to check on my appointment. During our discussions, he talked to me about a Dr. Sharma who had returned from the United States with a PhD. He informed me that since the position of Professor of Genetics (PVS I) at Hissar Veterinary College was vacant, he had offered him the position. Dr. Sharma had been reluctant to accept, but used the offer as a bargaining chip for a better paying position in the federal government. I told the Assistant Secretary that I had to fulfill a five-year bond of service, which denied me the luxury of shopping around. He then said that he was still considering me for the post but had not yet made up his mind. Mr. Mahli advised me to wait and assured me that he would contact me as soon as the decision reached his office.

It was mid-July. Father and the whole family had moved to Kot Khera into a one-bedroom house lent by a friend of the family. With my arrival, our family now numbered 12: my wife and our six children, my sister Darshan (who was unemployed), my parents, and Muni, a cousin. These were very difficult days.

Almost half of the village was in ruins. The mud-walled dwellings, once occupied by Muslims, were dilapidated, some reduced to mounds while others had walk-through holes in the walls. It was a depressing sight. Heavy monsoon rains had turned the area around the village into a wide belt of ankle-deep mud. My daily routine was to walk Father's six head of cattle barefoot through this mud-belt to our well. There, I had to mow some hay with a sickle, cut into short pieces with a chopper, and feed the cattle throughout the day. At sunset, I brought them home for the night. Bibi and Rajinder worked even harder. First, they had to break dead branches from trees in our fields and drag them home to use as firewood for cooking. Then, they spent the better part of the day collecting weeds, such as dandelions and mustard, for our supper. The menu and routines were the same, day after day.

All this time, the Assistant Secretary was stalling on my appointment. He knew that he held the upper hand, as the bond prohibited me applying elsewhere. I had no choice and no income. Bibi, with whom I always had a profound rapport, could hardly understand what was going on inside me. I had left Paris with so much hope of moving forward, but instead, I was losing ground and was constantly threatened by dark clouds of depression. As the waiting period dragged on, so did my feelings of hopelessness and despair.

During the hot summer, whenever it appeared that it would not rain at night, the family slept on the roof where it was cooler and breezier. The roof was quite spacious and enclosed by a three-foot red brick wall. Almost every evening, I would see an owl perched on this wall about 20 feet away from my bed, looking in our direction. He was quite fearless and would spend most of the night there. I was struck by this peculiar aberration, since the owl is a nocturnal bird of prey native to wooded areas. Its presence in a populated district, according to north Indian convictions, was an omen of bad luck.

An incident that happened at the end of my fellowship tenure in Mukteswar was still fresh in my mind. One afternoon, I had been chased by a small flock of blackbirds that circled above my head clamoring. They had been so vicious that I had to run for shelter. This quirky experience had been followed a month later by my troubles with Mr. Dhanda and my subsequent failure in my MVSc examinations. I dismissed the owl sighting as a freak coincidence. I had never been superstitious, nor did I believe in the occult. Nevertheless, the owl's lonely perch at the same place on the roof, night after night, made me wonder.

After two months, I could not wait any longer. I went back to see Mr. Mahli. He had just received a letter from the Assistant Secretary giving his decision that I could not be appointed directly. No reason was given. He was the same bureaucrat who, a few months earlier, had appointed Dr. Sharma to a higher ranking professor's position. However, in my case, he had needed two and a half months to refuse my appointment to the lower ranking position of assistant disease investigation officer. Dr. Sharma and I both had equivalent qualifications; the only difference was that I had more experience and a brighter academic career. The Assistant Secretary had acted with a double standard. I could only grin and bear the stinging effect of the news.

Mr. Mahli then called Mr. P.N. Nanda, Principal of the Veterinary College and asked if he could use an instructor. Mr. Nanda replied, "Yes, please send him to me at the college straight away." I had no choice but to march down that path that would be so devastating to my future. I knew that I would live to regret it. It was like trying to build a castle on shifting sand. Dejectedly, I started as an instructor, VAS grade, with a starting salary of RS100, the same salary at which I was first hired in July 1952. I felt like an inmate unjustly sentenced to serve five years in poverty because I had dared hope for a better life for myself and my family through higher education.

The College Principal

I came directly from the Director's office to Hissar and went straight to the Principal's office. I reported for duty on September 19, 1958. Mr. Nanda, serious and poised, told me that I was to work as an Instructor in the Pathology and Bacteriology Section.

The In-Charge of the Pathology and Bacteriology Section, Mr. Piara Singh Sahi and another demonstrator, Mr. Dharam Sarup Kalra (both were former teachers of mine), as well as the rest of the staff made me feel at home. I received a special welcome from my old college buddies, Onkar Singh Atwal, Ram Prakash Saini, and others who updated me on many recent developments at the college. They told me that Mr. Nanda had made many changes but that most were cosmetic. He had not had much success initiating research since he himself had no prior experience in this area and staff members were not willing to take on extra duties without extra pay. However, Mr. Nanda did have good intentions. He even gave out a step-by-step "recipe" on how to do research.

One night, my friends told me about Mr. Nanda's monthly teaching staff meetings where he gave details on his recipe. At the first meeting, he had stressed a need for reference cards which, according to him, were the main ingredients in research. These were to be used to jot down the main points of a research article after carefully reading at least one article a month. This process of reviewing articles and recording their main points was to be repeated. Research is about hard work, he would tell them, and researchers had to keep on trying until one day in a sacred moment something divine and magical would bring on a sudden new self-awareness. A researcher's mind would then be turned on, thereby stimulating a new idea. They would, then, put the idea in practice with a suitably devised experiment. There you are! Up and running and already researching!

I was told that everybody listened carefully, vowing to cooperate fully. Some even thought that the method was cool. When everyone flashed their newly bought reference cards at the second meeting, Mr. Nanda expressed great satisfaction with their good start. At the third meeting, everybody again waved reference cards; only this time they were filled in. Mr. Nanda was most enthusiastic about the progress of his mission. But, at subsequent meetings, his enthusiasm began to fade when nobody offered new ideas.

At the last meeting, Mr. Gopal Singh, Professor of Anatomy, talking from his long illustrious teaching experience, dealt a treacherous blow to Mr. Nanda's research mission. My friends related to me how he had pointed out, quite proudly of course, that a liver is a liver, a kidney is a kidney, and he had never seen a change in their size or shape to speak of. Therefore, there was hardly anything to research in anatomy. Mr. Nanda could not come up with a plausible refuting argument. More and more staff sided with the Professor of Anatomy and expressed somewhat similar philosophical views. Then, to Mr. Nanda's dismay, staff members collectively concluded that there was no reason for research in most of the subjects taught in a veterinary college. This action heralded a death knell to Mr. Nanda's vision.

Mr. Nanda's foray into research and the resulting fiasco as well as the anatomy professor's discursive comments had provided a heyday for jokes and numerous anecdotes, which they were only too eager to share with me. On a serious note, many asked how Mr. Nanda had managed to pull the wool over the Hon. Kairon's eyes, a man known for his perspicacity and astute judgment of human nature. I listened but decided to reserve judgment since I wanted to form my own unbiased opinion of Mr. Nanda. I needed to tread carefully in my dealings with the Principal, for he could do me a lot of good, but could also do a lot of damage. I had a career ahead of me and a large family to look after.

My Insubordination

I requested one day's casual leave to add on to the coming weekend to get my clothes, bedding etc. from home, which Mr. Nanda readily allowed. I reached Kot Khera in the rain, which was quite heavy at times because of an unusually long monsoon season that year. The area around Kot was flooded, at places knee-deep. The weather forced me to extend my leave another day. Finally, the rain stopped, and my daughter, Surinder, and I left for the railway station, wading half a mile through flood water. I had already missed a day of work, which no one thought was a grave matter. I put in a routine request for an extra day's leave through my Professor of Pathology to whom my absence should have mattered most. But, he passed it on to the Principal with a recommendation that the leave be sanctioned. This was a mere formality, or so I thought!

I was called to the Principal's office, where Mr. Nanda proceeded to interrogate me about the reason for my absence. After listening to the details, he said that his instincts in judging humans were sharp and that, in his dealings with veterinary assistants, he had heard all kinds of excuses to get out of awkward situations. He didn't believe a word that I said. I know that he expected me to stand before him, head bowed, eyes sheepishly lowered in a posture suggestive of an apology, and offer absolutely no contradictory statement. This was abhorrent to my sense of self-respect. Instead, I stood up and looked straight into his eyes and uttered my disagreement, which he interpreted as a sign of defiance and insubordination.

Mr. Nanda's comments, although inappropriate, were enough to raise concerns regarding the dignity of his office. I thought that, with time, the incidence would fade from his memory. But it didn't. At the annual assessment of employee performance, he made a red ink entry in my service book that I was insubordinate. I feared that such an entry would jeopardize my career and, therefore, put in an appeal to expunge the unfair and biased comment. The appeal was rejected, which was not surprising, since the management that ran the administration was the same one that dealt with appeals and grievances.

The Disease Investigation Officer, Radhey Mohan Sharma, was polite and courteous, but devious and cliquish in his affiliations. He was always cordial when we met face to face, but he was known for spreading gossip. Soon after I started at the Veterinary College, a close friend of mine told me that Mr. Mohan was circulating information about a meeting that he had with Dr. Lépine on his way back to India from England. Dr. Lépine, he claimed, had told him that I had performed poorly in his laboratory. When I confronted Mr. Mohan, he confirmed having seen Dr. Lépine and repeated his negative comments about me. I then asked him when exactly he had returned. He replied, "end of October 1956." "At that time," I said, "I was still in India. In fact, I did not even reach the Pasteur Institute until mid-December 1956. How could Dr. Lépine have given you his opinion without even knowing me?" Caught in his lies, Mr. Mohan stood there indifferent, unrepentant, and shameless. He had a direct line with Mr. Nanda, and his venom had already done irreparable damage to my career.

Over the next few months, I studied structural microscopic changes in the brain and spinal cords of sheep and goats affected with the so-called "lumbar paralysis," which occasionally swept through the flocks of Punjab's Breeding Farm at Hissar exacting a heavy toll. The changes and its reported symptoms were indistinguishable from those of Mad Cow Disease – a disease that was to become a matter of great concern to the western world in the year 2001. I sent a manuscript describing the changes in detail to the *Journal of Veterinary Science and Animal Husbandry*, whose editor sent it for review to Mr. Nanda. He, on expert advice from Mr. Mohan, recommended that the manuscript be rejected. Another journal, the *Indian Veterinary Journal*, accepted it readily without any reservation and published it in November 1959. This incident, in my mind, revealed the true level of Mr. Nanda's commitment to research.

Meanwhile, the lumbar paralysis, to use Mr. Nanda's expression, really "turned" me on. I suspected that the causal agent was a virus. During my two months' holidays in the summer of 1959, I went, at my own expense, to the Virus Laboratory in Poona, near Bombay. The laboratory was a leader in research on virus-induced infections of the human central nervous system. Their methods were equally applicable to virus infections in sheep and goats. I learned their fairly complicated techniques, which I typed and compiled in the form of a volume.

On my return, I talked briefly about my experience at Poona and showed Mr. Nanda the book. He kept turning the pages with his left hand, stroking his cigarette on the ashtray with his right, and nervously muttering "interesting, interesting." I couldn't figure out what was interesting – turning the pages or stroking the cigarette.

Fond Memories of Veterinary College

When I started as an instructor, the college campus was still under construction. Except for a few day students, all others lived on the campus, as did most of the staff. Students and teachers, despite living close to one another, had limited social contact and interacted only during lectures or practical workshops. Teachers believed that distance was necessary in order to command respect, a belief based on "familiarity breeds contempt." That belief, however, began to change, and one who showed respect by staying aloof was thought to be shy or lacking self-confidence.

About half of the 26 or so teaching staff were professors, and the rest were instructors. Most of the instructors had been my college mates and good friends. We all lived together in two rows of houses. We met frequently, and, collectively, we were involved with a large number of students. Onkar Atwal, Milkha Brar, and Lachman Hundle were good field hockey players who coached a college hockey team. Ram Prakash Saini, Harpal Bal, and I prepared a soccer team while Balbir Brar organized track and field events. We took our teams to several out-of-town tournaments. The students along with some of the instructors staged theatrical performances, satirical skits, and variety shows with dances, songs, and comedy acts. Onkar, who was known for his melodious voice, arranged sing along chorus shows.

We also created a Bhangra troupe who performed the popular traditional folk dance from Punjab's farming community. The dance is marked by vigorous body movements and loud music, backed by pounding drum beats. Its popularity is due to the gaiety, joy, brightness, and animation that it generates in the audience. Most of Bhangra's mesmerizing effects draw from theatrical and choreographic reenactment of farming activities, rich costumes, and buildup of momentum. Our performances drew crowds, and encores were the norm.

The many rehearsals and team sports connected us to a lot of students, and, directly and indirectly, we touched the heart of many. We discussed human values as fundamental tools for the health of a society and how being a good veterinarian was as important as being an honest person and a responsible citizen. Not once did we forget that our commitment to education was central in our lives. We believed that teachers had to open a dialogue with students and that serving them was our main and foremost role. We were there not only to teach science, but also to provide guidance on a number of complex issues such as morality and social justice. We often heard that we had made history. Some students even claimed that we were their role models. I treasure the memories from that period of my life.

Sadly, as time went by, the intellectual climate at the Veterinary College became more and more inhospitable. Most of us, if not all, migrated one by one to the United States, Canada, or Australia. Roughly 20 years after leaving India for good, Onkar returned to Hissar and stayed in the guest house at the Veterinary College campus. Many students came by to say hello and see him in person. They told him that they had heard a lot about him and his colleagues, and that to that day we were still very much alive in the students' memories.

Chapter 15: Hard Times Return

Tough Choices

Upon resuming my duties at the Veterinary College, I had taken Surinder with me to Hissar, where she started her university education in a government college. In August 1959, college authorities provided me with a two-and-a-half room house on campus rent-free. I brought the rest of my family to Hissar, thus relieving my parents once and for all of the responsibility of looking after them. Except for Nickky, all the children were in school or college; expenses for tuition, food, and clothing were high. I could not give them enough to eat. A friend from Khalsa College, Katha Singh, was farming close by. One day, he brought us a 60 kg bag of lentils to help us out. My professional degrees, skill, and hard work were proving to be worthless in providing the basic necessities for my family.

I tried hard to reestablish a rapport with my children and spent as much time with them as I could, especially with Nickky, Jyoti, and Awtar, who were still very young. Nickky would sit on my belly while I would be lying down, and she would ask me to sing for her. She would ask me over and over to sing more and more songs.

Our family was a democracy of some sort. I was a figure of authority, but quite flexible and reasonable. I respected my children and did not impose meaningless schedules or strictures. All of them were resilient, and each had his or her very own personality. They never posed a problem. Of course, they quarreled with each other, as is normal for children. They were bright, successful in their studies, and had developed good ethics and work habits. They pretty much grew up on their own, but I never forgot my responsibilities to them. I was also growing anxious about their future and whether I would ever be able to provide for them.

A competition was coming up for the position of assistant disease investigation officer, which I wanted badly. Most of the promotions in the Veterinary Department were by open competition through the Public Service Commission. For each opening, the Commission Chairman appointed a Selection Committee consisting of three members, two PSC employees and a co-opted technical member who was recommended by the Secretary of the

Department of Agriculture. The Secretary generally recommended either the Director of the Veterinary Department or the Principal of the Veterinary College, depending on who the selected candidate would work for. Obviously, Mr. Nanda would be the committee's technical member since the position was under his administration.

I was also aware that there were no standard or consistent criteria for the selection of candidates. Questions asked during an interview varied between candidates and were sometimes irrelevant and quite often discriminatory. Interviews were difficult if the authorities did not favor a particular candidate. Because of his technical expertise, the co-opted member invariably prevailed in getting the favored person in. Due to my recent difficulties with Mr. Nanda, I had strong doubts of winning the competition.

A friend and colleague, Harpal Bal, happened to be a close relative of the Chief Minister of Punjab, the Hon. Kairon. I asked Harpal to arrange a hearing with the Minister so that I could air my concerns. Harpal and I spent the night at the Minister's residence, and the next day, the Hon. Kairon took us to his office in his limousine. From there, he called the Minister of Agriculture, Giani Kartar Singh.

I presented my case succinctly, stating that I was the most highly qualified professional in the Punjab Veterinary Department, yet the lowest paid because of a five-year service bond that I had signed under duress. I asked the ministers to release me from this bond or else arrange for my salary to be commensurate with my experience and qualifications. The Chief Minister waved his hand at Giani Kartar Singh, who then took me to his office. He called the Secretary of Agriculture, Mr. K.S. Narang, and told him to listen to what I had to say and report back to him. I ended up with the Secretary in his office. Mr. Narang lit into me for going to higher authorities and threatened me with disciplinary action. He boasted that he was the boss and not the Minister or Chief Minister, since they came and went with elections like migratory birds.

When he saw that I was not moved by his silly threats, he changed his strategy. He became infuriated with my complacence and promised that his wrath would bring forth the worst retaliation. I commended him for having done not too badly, even when he had not been so angry. He had, after all, succeeded in keeping me hostage at a humiliating salary with no possibility of improvement. I got up to leave. He urged me to sit down.

Sensing my stiffened resolve and probably fearful of the Minister's backlash, Mr. Narang beat a hasty retreat. We should all work together, he said, to make the 20th century India's century. (I had no comments on his clairvoyance.) Because our country is riddled with poverty, he added, we should be creative and innovative, working selflessly with a spirit of sacrifice. I replied, "Sir, you earn about Rs2,000 a month. If you are willing to work for Rs100 a month, we could both be doing a national service; in fact, I would welcome that." He was not impressed. I reminded him that I had sought out the Hon. Chief Minister for a wrong to be redressed and not to engage in counterproductive discussions. I again got up to leave. Again, he asked me to sit down – this time politely.

What did I want? he asked. "I want you to appoint me to the post of Assistant Disease Investigation Officer right away and assure me that the forthcoming competition will be fair," adding that Mr. Nanda would not be an appropriate technical member of the Selection Committee. I left his office a half hour later with a letter appointing me assistant disease investigation officer. A few weeks later, I was selected by the Public Service Commission, thus making me permanent.

Honorable Giani Kartar Singh

I had known the Honorable Giani Kartar Singh, then the elected Minister of Agriculture, for at least ten years. He was from the District of Hoshiarpur. The title "Giani" is a common form of address reserved for someone who has graduated with a Diploma of Giani in Punjabi language. He was a political phenomenon, selfless, humble, simple, highly respected, and without any desire for material possessions. He had an uncanny skill in political maneuvering, changing Punjab's Chief Ministers at will and, thus, was nicknamed "Kingmaker."

As a minister, he lived in a government-provided furnished ministerial mansion with his total worldly possession of two sets of clothes – white *kacha* and shirt, and blue turban – all made of homespun cotton. He wore one set while the other dried on the clothesline. He lived with his sister; both were unmarried. His sister managed the house with a budget just big enough to cover the cost of hosting the many visiting party workers and people from his home constituency.

When his government was defeated in a vote of non-confidence, he had been visiting with a friend. He merely sent a message to his sister instructing her to vacate the mansion and to meet him bringing his clothes from the clothesline. His simple nonchalant and gracious manner of moving out of the house that had been home for several years made headlines.

He was meticulously honest and, to my knowledge, never accepted kickbacks or was involved in any unsavory dealings. He ardently promoted Punjabi, never speaking in English. In 1958 when he was invited to close a three-day track and field event at the Veterinary College in Hissar, he gave his address in Punjabi. After saying "I declare the...," he stopped as if searching for the right Punjabi word for "track and field." Unable to come up with one, he continued "What do you call that? Well, well, whatever you call it, it is now closed." Everyone laughed, and the closing event became table talk for several days.

I had the opportunity to meet with him twice. Both times I felt I was in the presence of a legend. He always wore a faint smile, and his voice was gentle and soft. His expression and tone of voice never changed, making it impossible to judge his mood. He was a man of reason who worked with conviction and vision for the good of the community. He was a great man.

In Trouble Again

I took up my new position on October 3, 1959 and immediately set about equipping my two-room laboratory. My colleagues had bought the latest and most expensive equipment from catalogues, more out of rivalry than need, which they proudly displayed. I had good relations with all of them, and they readily lent me what I needed. In very little time, I had a functioning tissue culture facility. I bought mice, guinea pigs, and rabbits, bred them in the vacant animal colony building, and concentrated my research on rabies and foot and mouth disease.

I successfully grew kidney cells on the flat surface inside glass whisky bottles since laboratory flasks were not available in India. I knew of only one other Indian laboratory culturing cells in vitro, and they were getting all their equipment and funding from American universities. Because I lacked the proper equipment, I had to modify procedures, making use of what was available. Within two years, I had published two research papers in an American journal and two more in an Indian journal. In addition, two postgraduate students qualified their MVSc degrees under my guidance. But Mr. Nanda was not at all pleased that research was finally being carried out in his institution. He remained cold and indifferent.

In 1960, I applied for the newly created position of assistant professor of pathology. The Selection Committee, with Mr. Nanda as technical member, rejected my candidacy and selected, instead, a colleague and earlier co-instructor, Dharam Sarup Kalra. He held a BVSc, ten years teaching experience, and no scientific publications. On the other hand, I had master's and doctoral degrees, six years of research, two years of teaching, and six research publications. Mr. Nanda had successfully set up Mr. Kalra as the future professor of pathology, stalling my career at the same time.

My routine at work was to go to the local slaughterhouse at 5 am every Monday to collect goat kidneys and blood, bring them to the laboratory, and initiate the culturing process. I would go home at about 8:30 for breakfast and return to the laboratory around 9:30 to continue the culturing process to completion. One Monday morning when I returned from breakfast, I was surprised to see Mr. Nanda nervously pacing back and forth in front of my laboratory. On seeing me, he frowned, pointed to his wristwatch, and demanded to know why I was half an hour late for work. I gave him the reason and then proceeded to impart a lot more information than he had come for. I showed him the cultures and acquainted him with my ongoing research. He never said a word. He was obviously disappointed in having failed to find fault. Soon after, Mr. Nanda's contract expired. There was no customary farewell ceremony at the college, and none of the staff members bade him goodbye.

My earlier MVSc guide, Mr. Dhanda, Mr. Nanda, and many others considered themselves members of the ruling elite. They were convinced of their superiority, just as they were of the inferiority of their subordinates. They belonged to the outdated British colonial era which dictated a culture of servitude. Holding on to power was their main focus. They created a culture of flattery and favoritism without any vision. In India's post-independent democratic times, they adapted poorly, showing equally poor judgment and certainly no leadership in free expression. Above all, they abhorred and resisted change with tenacity and held on to old ideas with obstinacy. History has shown that the relative difference in progress between civilizations depends on their readiness to change, adapt to new ideas, cumulate knowledge, and make inventions. A civilization's readiness to change profoundly affects its people, their thoughts, feelings, and conduct.

A Professorship, At Last

In 1961, Nigeria became an independent nation within the Commonwealth of Nations. Immediately after independence, British officers in the Nigerian Civil Service resigned en masse, creating a vacuum in almost every department. The Indian Government, in a spirit of friendliness, allowed the Nigerian Public Service Commission to recruit Indian nationals who were willing to work in Nigeria. The Commission came to India to interview personnel for many positions, including that of principal of the Veterinary College and a disease investigation officer.

There were 31 candidates for these two positions, including me, waiting to be interviewed at New Delhi's Ashoka Hotel. The Selection Committee consisted of two members of the Nigerian Commission and the Secretary of Indian Foreign Affairs. I was the first candidate to be interviewed. The Secretary opened the interview with a volley of questions that were not to my liking. He asked, "Are you applying for the job with the permission of the Punjab Government? Are you aware that there are reprisals for contravening this requirement?" I answered, "Yes, I know about the reprisals and will fight them if I have to." "Do you know why you have not been gainfully employed by the Punjab Government?" he asked. I said, "This is a question for the Punjab Government to answer, not me."

The Secretary tried his best to portray me as insubordinate and troublesome. I responded that I was an exemplary employee according to PEPSU's annual assessments and that the Punjab Government had been unjust in their reports. At that point, the Secretary let the matter rest. Questions from the other two commission members were banal. The interview ended on a note of pessimism.

To my surprise, I received a letter about a week later from the Nigerian Commission announcing that I had been selected Disease Investigation Officer. Tickets and a check for traveling expenses were to be sent upon receipt of a medical report. I was overjoyed. I immediately sent back the required health certificate and chest x-ray. The very next day, I received a telegram from Mr. Narang asking me to come to see him at once at his office in Chandigarh. Apparently, something had transpired between the Secretary of Foreign Affairs and Mr. Narang. What it was, I will never know. My selection had somehow precipitated a crisis. During the meeting, Mr. Narang threatened me with disciplinary action for not having applied through proper government channels and stated emphatically that he would stop my posting to Nigeria.

I didn't want to be on the defensive anymore. I also knew that he could not stop my departure. I told him point blank that his threats were empty and that upbraiding and threatening me with disciplinary action was pointless. The Nigerian job offer had given me leverage, and I didn't hesitate to tell him that he needed to work on his communications skills. Gradually, he mellowed, becoming conciliatory. I was not misled by this change in attitude; I knew it was not a change of heart. He desperately wanted me to refuse the Nigerian offer and stay on at the laboratory.

"What can I do that would convince you to stay?" he asked. He wanted a letter from me addressed to the Nigerian Commission expressing my inability to go to Nigeria. I told him that he could only get such a letter, after I was appointed professor of pathology and bacteriology, first directly and later by the Public Service Commission. He told me that with my qualifications and experience there should not be a problem with the Commission's selection process. An hour later, I had a letter appointing me professor. I took over the charge on January 27, 1962. Regrettably, I had not had the savvy to bargain for a higher pay scale. Ironically, the promotion failed to bring any significant financial relief to me and my family, since I was no longer entitled to free accommodation. I now had to pay rent for a house two miles from campus.

A Difficult Decision

In 1960, research on lumbar paralysis in sheep was in full swing at the Hissar's sheep breeding farm. Mr. P.C. Sekariah, an investigator from Mukteswar's Veterinary Research Institute, came to the farm to study the disease. That same afternoon, he sent a messenger from the clinic in the animal breeding farm asking me to go and see him. He pointed to the microscope that had a slide prepared from cerebrospinal fluid of a sheep suffering from lumbar paralysis and said, "There it is, the agent that causes lumbar paralysis." Lo and behold, there were live worms!

In my studies of some 46 sheep, I had never before seen a single worm either in the cerebrospinal fluid or in stained sections prepared from fixed brain tissues. But, Mr. Sekariah had allegedly found the worms in the very first animal he had examined. He packed up and left the next day, his mission accomplished. After his departure, I examined cerebrospinal fluid from a few more sick sheep, but never again saw the enigmatic worm. I wondered, *Where had Mr. Sekariah's worms really come from?*

Mr. Sekariah also tried to solve the mystery of another disease, Toxoplasmosis. He, with P.G. Pande and P.K. Ramachandran of the

Veterinary Research Institute, published a paper reporting highly significant findings on Toxoplasmosis in the 1961 *Journal of Infectious Diseases* (vol. 108, pp. 68 74). An American professor and expert on Toxoplasmosis was intrigued with their findings, so much so that he came to Mukteswar. His surprise visit heralded bad news for the scientists. The professor requested their raw data, and after scrutiny found nothing that substantiated their claim. Before flying back to the U.S., he stopped in New Delhi for a visit with Mr. Nehru, India's Prime Minister. The visit triggered an investigation of plagiarism against the authors by the Government of India. The government report was damaging for several Veterinary Institute researchers. Mr. Sekariah was dismissed. The *Journal of Infectious Diseases'* Editorial Board published an apology on the opening page of its May-June 1961 issue (Vol. 108, No. 3).

Reverberations were felt by scientists throughout the nation, sending a wake-up call to reviewers and editors of scientific journals. Some of us who were engaged in veterinary research felt a responsibility to follow moral imperatives and discourage the reporting of fudged or fake data.

At the end of February 1962, the federal government organized a three-day annual meeting in Madras, chaired by the Director of the Indian Veterinary Institute. All disease investigation officers and assistants, as well as professors of pathology and of parasitology from all veterinary colleges in India, were invited to present their research findings. Mr. Mohan, our Disease Investigation Officer, presented a study on a recent outbreak of an infectious disease in sheep at Hissar Animal Breeding Farm. In his paper, he claimed to have identified a parasite similar to one that had caused an outbreak in Australian sheep the previous year. In the course of his research, he claimed to have used an ultracentrifuge at the Indian Veterinary Institute.

I questioned Mr. Mohan's findings since his paper had come up short on many counts. From September 1958 on, I had been actively involved with all the sheep flocks at the Animal Breeding Farm – first when doing research on sheep's lumbar paralysis and, later, on sheep and goat diseases. I had never seen such an outbreak. Further, Mr. Mohan had no photographs of the alleged parasites, and the Indian Veterinary Research Institute did not have the type of centrifuge Mr. Mohan claimed to have used. On hearing my questions, Mr. Mohan stood dumbfounded. He had no answers. The chairman, who had been Head of the Parasitology Division before becoming director, confirmed that the Indian Veterinary Institute had no ultracentrifuge.

Rebuttal, or posing embarrassing questions, was not customary in these meetings. A listener either accepted or rejected the results quietly, and any deviation from this norm failed to find favor with the audience. As a consequence, I was subjected to very unpleasant repercussions. Only four researchers appreciated my efforts. The remaining participants were mostly cold and indifferent, some even treating me as an outcast. Their tacit approval of falsified data ran against the very basic precepts of science. I could not continue working in this kind of atmosphere. I had encountered enough difficulties in my career. I started thinking seriously about leaving India for good.

Indian society, I thought, was in a quandary. Top officials of the federal and provincial bureaucracy, the public at large, and the Congress Party all interacted intrinsically, thus generating a characteristic pattern of social behavior. The intransigent top bureaucracy demanded loyalty, flattery, and obedience verging on servitude from its lower ranks who, in turn, made similar demands from the public. Many public officials were power hungry, not accountable to anyone, and were driven by anything but logic. The public by and large was submissive and tried to appease the authoritarian bureaucracy in order to gratify their own self-interests. The rank and file of the governing Congress Party made hardly any effort to create a government that would work for the public good and serve the public interest. Instead, they lobbied for aggrieved individuals, irrespective of merit. They constantly interfered with the decisions of top officials. Disappointed, the public turned more and more to politicians for redress and favors.

Throughout my career, I had refused to submit to demeaning and humiliating treatment, I had refused to stoke a superior's vanity for the purpose of advancement. I did not possess political finesse, nor did I conform to society's norms. I just did not fit in, nor did my father before me. He had ended up a failure. I wanted to be a success, in spite of all efforts to push me down. I had been dealt so many disappointments throughout the years. In spite of having faced arrogant authorities with defiance, audacity, and cynicism, I had done well enough, climbing to the top-ranking permanent post of professor (PVS I). I was confident that I could continue to progress without compromising myself, but I also knew what it would cost me in terms of time and effort. I was not too keen on living my life in a continuous fight with the Indian bureaucracy.

My poverty-ridden childhood, with food always a primary concern, had taught me to make do with less. I could have lived a simple life, but I had a family, a wife, and six children. The children had to have a good education. I wanted a better life for them. My earnings could not buy them that. I also had four daughters; their weddings and dowry loomed large in my thoughts. All these worries helped seal my decision to leave India. I was heavy-hearted, for it was a very difficult decision.

Chapter 16: Postdoctoral Training

Life in the U.S.

My mind made up, I began writing to American universities and research institutes that were active in viral studies (22 in all), applying for a research posting. In March 1962, I received a letter from the Department of Virology and Epidemiology of Baylor University in Houston, Texas, offering me a Fulbright Postdoctoral Fellowship. I was thrilled at the opportunity of studying in the U.S. I quickly wrote back accepting their offer. The university subsequently sent me an air ticket, $100 traveling money, and a J-1 non-migrant visa. In August, I received a second offer of a postdoctoral assistantship from the University of Illinois in Urbana, Illinois, which I declined.

In October, the Governor of Punjab sanctioned a 195-day leave, 75 days earned leave plus 120 days at half pay for higher training. Since all my travel and living expenses were to be paid from the Fellowship, I thought that obtaining the Permission (P) Form of the State Bank of India to leave the country would be a walk in the park. This P form was used to determine whether or not an Indian national going abroad had financial backing adequate for the duration of the trip. A candidate had to submit the completed form in person, along with supporting documents and passport, to a clerk in the State Bank of India in New Delhi. The clerk then directed the papers to one of two bank officials who would review the information and make a decision.

Hordes of candidates waited in the hall outside. I could see through the open office doors that each official had large stacks of papers which were getting higher with the unending flow of documents from the clerk. The official would take a perfunctory look at each document and make a decision that appeared, at least to me, instinctual rather than one based on documentary evidence.

After waiting about two hours, a stack was brought out and placed on a large table outside the hall. I located mine. It had come back with "permission · not granted." I was crushed. Quickly, I had to think of some way to get this decision reversed. I recalled that the father of one of my students worked in

149

the State Bank of India. After some thought, his family name came to me, and I started my search. I eventually found the man in the same building. After listening to my plight, he took me back to the hall and got me to fill out another P form. He took the completed form to one of the officials and got my earlier refusal changed to "permission granted." I breathed a sigh of relief, but I was not surprised that the decision could be altered.

At the time of my departure, Surinder, Jag, and Balbir were attending the local government college, while Awtar, Jyoti, and Nickky were in school. They were all doing very well, and I had no worry on their account. I bought a buffalo-cow from a colleague. (I paid him for it once I got to the U.S.) It would provide enough milk and butter for my growing family. Rajinder would receive my full salary for two and a half months and half of my salary for four months. Surinder, Jag, and Balbir worried about what it would be like when I was gone, whereas Awtar, Jyoti, and Nickky were too young to understand. About half an hour before my actual departure, Awtar, who was then 11 years old, decided that he did not want to wait around. He said goodbye and went to play cricket. Rajinder was extremely depressed and sad. I feared an uncertain future.

On November 4, 1962, I took an overnight flight from New Delhi to Paris, where I spent the day meeting with friends at the Pasteur Institute. Another overnight flight brought me to New York, and a connecting flight took me to Houston in the evening. This would be my new home for the next year. The following day, I started working at the Virus Laboratories of Baylor University. My professor had rented a bachelor apartment for me, which was within walking distance of the university, just opposite the football stadium of Rice University.

I missed my family a lot, and within a week, I developed a terrible feeling of loneliness that plunged me into a state of depression and anxiety. I started experiencing dizzy spells. My head would whirl, and I had a tendency to lose my balance, especially when I made a sudden movement. The symptoms gradually disappeared. I found out later that I had had a "silent heart attack," which remained undetected until 1979. I wrote to Rajinder and the children regularly. My fellowship at Houston paid me $376 a month after deductions. Out of that, I sent home about one-third, which was sufficient for the family to live comfortably.

At work, I didn't have the luxury to pick and choose my projects. I was assigned to complete the research initiated by a postdoctoral fellow whose term had ended on my arrival. I finished the project and published the findings in the *Journal of Immunology* in the form of a paper which became one of my highly cited publications. This was the only bright event of my stay in Houston.

With the dizziness gone, I was again full of vigor. A friend of mine who was also a postdoctoral fellow, Guy Van, offered to teach me how to drive. He had a Volkswagen and gave me driving lessons until I was ready for the road test. I bought an old Volkswagen and resumed playing soccer. I also learned how to play tennis and made many friends. I was finally coming out of my shell.

I didn't want to go back to India. There, I would have to live on hope alone, which could only suit an eternal optimist. I bought a typewriter and started looking for work. I wrote to universities and institutions across Canada and the United States. It seemed as if I was always typing applications, and the letter carrier was forever bringing me letters of regret. But, three institutions seemed to be interested in hiring me. That gave me hope. Later though, they reneged, and I wondered why. It never occurred to me at that time that my J-1 non-immigrant visa was the cause; it was restrictive, limiting my stay in the U.S. to a maximum of two years. This only dawned on me much later when I was about to leave.

Keeping in mind that I might have to return to India, I applied on August 9 for the advanced increments due to me in view of my postdoctoral training. I didn't receive a reply. I followed up on September 8 and still did not get a response. In October, I wrote again – this time asking for an extension of my leave without pay for three and a half more months. My previous leave of absence was due to expire on November 30.

Meanwhile, I found out that the Public Service Commission of Canada was looking for a pathologist for its Food and Drug Directorate in Ottawa. I applied for the post on October 24. On November 5, the Commission contacted Mrs. Heather, a co-worker at Baylor University and one of my referees. On November 27, they wrote that the Selection Board was reviewing my qualifications. It further asked me to stay connected, were there a change in address.

Time was running out. My term as postdoctoral fellow expired on December 23, 1963. I left Houston on Christmas Eve with an air ticket to New Delhi, $600, and high hopes of landing the pathologist job in Ottawa. I decided to wait in New York City at the YMCA's William Sloane House.

I paid $3 a day for my room. I immediately applied for immigration to Canada and received an encouraging letter. The Immigration Branch of Alberta would make an effort to develop an alternative opportunity if the federal government failed in its job offer at Ottawa.

I got my visa extended to March 10 and sent $100 to my family in Hissar explaining my difficulties. I was getting low on cash. It was a nailbiting period filled with intense anxiety and suspense. I lived from moment to moment, desperately waiting. My only other alternative was to fly back to India, and that thought was even more stressful. It seemed to me that I was standing on the edge of an abyss.

My application to extend my leave was turned down by the Vice Chancellor. In his letter, he wrote, "The Vice-Chancellor of Punjab Agriculture University is pleased to refuse grant of extraordinary leave… absence of duty beyond 30.11.1963 shall be liable to disciplinary action." Interesting, isn't it? I sent in my resignation by return post.

Finally, a letter arrived, asking if I was interested in working as pathologist at the Food and Drug Directorate! The letter was dated February 10, but had gone to Houston and did not reach me in New York until February 20. This letter changed the course of my future, from one filled with continuous struggles to a much brighter one. It brought an end to the anxiety that had been plaguing me.

I immediately accepted by telephone and received the official offer by telegram on February 21. I requested permission from the Department of Citizenship and Immigration to enter Canada in anticipation of the completion of immigration formalities. I was granted permission on March 3, again by telegram. The next day in the afternoon, I landed at the Ottawa airport with $18.75 in my pocket, a few clothes, and a big dream.

Chapter 17: Canada: My New Home

The Food and Drug Directorate

To immigrate to Canada, I needed letters from the Indian government and from my father stating that they had no objections to my migration. Immigration officials also required medical certificates from my wife and children. The latter took some time to come, since Rajinder and the children had minor medical conditions that required lengthy treatment. I was granted landed immigrant status on October 13, 1967 and became a Canadian citizen on July 23, 1971.

On the morning of March 5, 1964, I reported for work as pathologist at the Food and Drug Directorate of the Department of National Health and Welfare, at Tunney's Pasture in Ottawa. My position was classified as Biologist 3 with an annual salary of $8,750.

I stayed in a room at the YMCA until I found an apartment. I lived on borrowed money until my first paycheck, eating sparsely at cheap restaurants and cafeterias. I wrote immediately to Rajinder, describing my new job, my apartment, and what Ottawa was like. I promised to send some money as soon as I got paid.

The Pathology section had three professionals: a biochemist, Dr. Stuart Wiberg, and two pathologists, Dr. Harold Grice (Duke), who was section head, and myself. In addition, the section had three technicians, but it did not have its own independent research projects because Dr. Grice was under instructions from higher authority to work for other researchers in the Directorate. He conducted postmortems on animals used in research, gross and microscopic study of tissues, including blood or hematology, and wrote reports of their findings for publication.

Two weeks in the job, Duke sent me to see Dr. Mannell. Dr. Mannell had asked for my help in a new investigation on the long-term effects of a certain pesticide in rats. I had met him a few days earlier when Duke was conducting postmortems on Dr. Mannell's rats. Dr. Mannell had watched from a distance holding a handkerchief over his mouth and nose. This struck me as somewhat odd behavior for a scientist involved in animal studies.

During our meeting, Dr. Mannell outlined his experiment which, briefly, was to feed 200 rats with a daily mix of pesticide and food at different concentrations. A group of 50 rats were to be killed every six months. I was to conduct complete postmortem examinations on all the rats and study a wide array of tissues for changes in their weight and structure. My contribution was a major part of the project. I knew that his technician would weigh out the pesticide for the different dietary concentrations and that the personnel of the animal colony would look after feeding the rats. I asked Dr. Mannell about his role in the study. He said that he would be the project leader – in other words, the senior author. He would supervise the whole project and prepare the manuscript for publication. I had heard that before. I didn't need to be supervised, and I also knew how to use the weighing balance. I suggested that, as a participant, he could perhaps investigate changes in certain enzymes of various tissues. He shrugged with indifference.

At the end of our meeting, I told him that I would welcome the opportunity of collaborating with him, provided that his contribution equaled mine. Our discussion ended on an uncompromising note. Duke was annoyed with me and reminded me that this was the type of work I had been hired to do. He was, however, very understanding and responsive to reason. He agreed with me that not only did a project have to be imaginative and pose a challenge, but its collaborators also should make equitable contributions. In that case, he said, I had to come up with a project of my own.

Pesticides and Thalidomide

Two events occurred in 1962, and their aftereffects had an important bearing on science and research. Unbeknownst to me at the time, these events would alter the course of my future in research.

The first was the publication of Rachel Carson's book, *Silent Spring*, which showed how humans had polluted their own environment with pesticides so that their very existence was threatened by disease and death. Carson's book had an enormous impact on scientists and politicians. It reinforced what environmentalists had been saying all along – that the use of pesticides had profound effects on birds and aquatic species. Organophosphates, especially DDT, were detrimental to human health. There were strong scientific opinions that, with the current state of limited knowledge on biological effects, it was imperative that governments regulate the use of pesticides and determine at what level these toxic chemicals could be allowed in the air, soil, water, and vegetables. Scientific studies on pesticides and other chemicals, including drugs, were needed to determine safe levels.

The second event, which was much more important, was the independent publications of Drs. W. McBride (1961) and W. Lens (1962). They reported the discovery of a human tragedy in the form of congenital birth defects produced by thalidomide, a recently marketed drug prescribed to women in early pregnancy to control morning sickness. Thalidomide caused severe birth defects of upper and lower limbs in more than 2,000 babies in Canada alone, and several thousands in Europe and Japan.

The infamous drug had escaped the government's scrutiny because regulators in western countries had required limited data on risk assessment and had sometimes allowed a chemical or drug to be marketed on the claim of safety alone. The determination of congenital defects produced by chemicals was then a part of multigenerational studies. Rats and mice were fed daily with diets containing different concentrations of a drug or chemical to be tested for three or more generations. Every morning, the females were examined for births, and the number of pups born the night before were examined and counted. This method had an inherent shortcoming – it overlooked the fact that some malformed pups may have died the night before and been cannibalized by the mother.

In the aftermath of the thalidomide tragedy, regulatory processing and law governing the commercial use of drugs and chemicals started to change. Suddenly, there was a strong need to devise new methods for the appraisal of the malformative (teratogenic) potential of chemicals, such as drugs, food additives, and food contaminants. Governments and their regulatory agencies, not wanting to be caught in the center of another thalidomide-like embarrassment, were faced with a new reality. Regulators could not do anything about the many commercially used chemicals that had sketchy data, but they could require teratology data on all new chemicals before they could be marketed. And they did.

To meet the challenge, the science of teratology started studying the effects of drugs on fetal development. There were lots of jobs and grant money but a shortage of personnel with appropriate scientific knowledge. Teratology was not yet a well-defined subject and was not studied at university. The money and jobs lured workers with backgrounds as diverse as chemistry, biochemistry, pharmacy, pharmacology, and genetics. Their zeal was hardly in doubt.

My Laboratory – a Hatchery

There were no standards for testing chemicals. It was not even known which animal specie would be most suitable in tests assessing human risk. The U.S. Food and Drug Administration (FDA) and the Canadian Food and Drug Directorate had similar mandates, which was to control human exposure to noxious chemicals, whether pesticides, food contaminants, or drugs. FDA scientists, McLaughlin *et al* had published in 1963 and 1964 that embryos developing in chicken eggs could be useful in assessing the toxic and birth defect inducing (teratogenic) potential of chemicals. Borrowing from this concept, I prepared a research proposal to explore the relevance of chick embryos, and added duck embryos as my own idea, for assessing the safety of pesticides. The Directorate, with Dr. J.C. Campbell at the helm, was most anxious to initiate research in this new area and readily approved the proposal.

But, there was a hitch. There was no budget. I needed eggs and an egg incubator. I found an incubator – a museum piece collecting dust – in storage at the Laboratory of Hygiene across the road from our building. It was a wooden cabinet with a capacity of no more than three dozen eggs. In preliminary tests, individual injections of EPN and Systox (insecticides) in duck eggs produced serious and permanent malformations in the ducklings. The Director, Duke, and many others in the building were impressed outright with these malformations. They were, in fact, very dramatic and aroused curiosity, reminding me of something I had seen when I was 12 years old – a live two-headed calf.

The incubator that I had required that each egg be rotated manually three to four times a day. Plus, it could not maintain the temperature at an acceptable range. It had no mechanism to regulate humidity which I solved by placing a pan of water inside. I had to find a better incubator. Upon scouring the laboratories in Ottawa, I discovered that Dr. Quinton LaHam of the Biology Department of the University of Ottawa had one, a free laboratory, and an $8,000 grant from the National Research Council. Dr. LaHam received me with open arms and placed his facilities at my disposal. He and I worked together for a year. I only showed my face at the Directorate to pick up my pay check. Quinton and I presented our results in March 1965 at the Fourth Annual Meeting of the Society of Toxicology held in Williamsburg, Virginia. I subsequently published three research papers (Khera and LaHam, 1965; Khera, LaHam, and Grice, 1965; Khera *et al*,

1966).

In the next budget year, there was lots of money available. I bought a state-of-the-art incubator-hatchery and eggs by the thousands. I injected 13 pesticides, each at three dose levels in duck and chick eggs during their four different stages of development. To be thorough, each experiment was repeated three times. The whole investigation required more than 17,000 eggs of each specie. My work place looked more like a hatchery than a laboratory!

The results of this study (Khera and Lyon, 1968) and others from different laboratories were reviewed (Khera and Clegg, 1969). The review showed that avian embryos had limited usefulness in assessing human safety. Embryonic responses in these species differed from those in mammals and were quite often exaggerated or not reproducible, probably because an avian embryo develops in isolation from the mother and placenta and, consequently, from its protective and detoxifying mechanisms. It grows in a "closed" system and lacks the ability to excrete an injected chemical. I closed my hatchery and moved on to mammals.

Safety Assessment of Chemicals

During the 1950s, the safety of drugs and chemicals for human reproduction was assessed from a three-generation reproduction study conducted mostly in mice or rats. These were the animals of choice for economy of space, ease of handling, housing, feeding, and other reasons. Most of the criteria or endpoints of reproduction were measured in quantitative terms and recorded for statistical analyses. These were libido, fertility, fertilization of ova, survival and growth of the fetus, delivery, and growth of offspring. Adverse effects on fetal development were evaluated from these reproduction studies.

Both the American and Canadian governments decreed in 1962 that two studies be added to the already mandatory three-generation study. The first was a study of the effects of chemicals and drugs on fertility in males and females over a span of one generation. The second was a study of birth defects in which animals were dosed during pregnancy and the term fetuses examined for viability, body weight, and malformations. The data from all three types of reproduction studies were analyzed in the same manner.

Animal studies were crucial then, and still are, in assessing the safety of chemicals. They provide the necessary data to set standards for human exposure to chemicals. The conduct of these studies is fairly technical and demands a know-how to collect data on a wide array of endpoints for the above three types of reproduction studies. The results are analyzed to determine that the adverse effects are genuine and that there is a dose showing no apparent adverse effect which is called no observed adverse effect level (NOAEL or NOEL). Under certain circumstances, if NOEL is not available, a low observed effect level (LOEL) is used.

A NOEL is divided by what is called a safety or risk factor to arrive at an Allowable Daily Intake (ADI) for humans, and a tolerance level for each of the various sources of human exposure such that a total amount contributed by each source does not exceed the ADI. The tolerance levels and ADI are calculated in parts per million (ppm). The latter is the amount of a chemical in its medium (body, body tissues, cereals, vegetables, etc.) and is customarily expressed on a weight-to-weight concentration in ppm.

The risk or safety factor is a numerical figure crudely estimated to compensate for three uncertainties in: (1) the prediction of safety for humans from animal data, (2) variations in sensitivity from animal to animal, and (3) individual variations in humans for which the use of the chemical is intended. The magnitude of the safety factor is determined arbitrarily and could be as high as 1,000.

There are, however, shortcomings in assessing the safety of a chemical. Many people presume that animal studies are completely reliable and provide clear answers as to whether or not a chemical is safe. The reality is that quite often animal studies produce conflicting data that is difficult to interpret. For instance, two or more animal species, even when tested with the same chemical, may give different results making it impossible to determine which of the specie is more suitable. These problems are further compounded by the arbitrarily determined safety factor which is based on questionable assumptions. In my opinion, it is important for lay people to understand that the regulatory agencies' public policy on risk assessment has these serious limitations.

Teratology Assessments – a Historical Account

Of the above three types of reproduction study, the teratology study is the main focus of the following section. Teratology is the study of defects that occur during the development of an embryo or fetus[8] and become apparent at birth or later. In 1960, there was no single method to evaluate chemicals for fetal effects acceptable to all investigators. The literature contained a constellation of methods, a whole gamut of ideas on evaluation of animal data, and several ways of measuring human safety from the data. There were contending and conflicting views, but few facts.

It became imperative to develop explicit methods to uncover a chemical's possible adverse effects on fetal development. A variety of methods were reported, and the only aspect agreed upon was dosing during pregnancy and examination of the term fetuses obtained by caesarian section. Scientists used different laboratory species, varying length of time for administering a chemical, and routes of administration as bizarre as vaginal application. There was no limit on how much of a drug could be given. A few malformed fetuses were all that was required to label a chemical teratogenic. Some studies went to the ridiculous extreme of showing that common table salt and sugar – at unrealistically high doses and under flawed experimental conditions – could cause adverse effects on a fetus. There was a common joke in teratology testing that it's not the drug that was being introduced to a mouse, but the mouse being introduced to a drug.

Early in the 1960s, nobody knew what the new findings meant or what an appropriate experimental design for extrapolating human safety was. The effect of toxicity on fetal development was a new branch of the science of teratology, and it was experiencing "growing pains." However, none of these studies stirred up public awareness or media support to have the chemicals banned by regulatory agencies until 1968.

Cyclamate and MSG

One study published in 1969 did hit a raw nerve. It was published in Japan and alleged that sodium cyclamate, the most widely used artificial sweetener, caused toxic effects on rat embryos. Dr. J.M. Verrett from the FDA showed defective skeletons of chick embryos from eggs injected with the sweetener. She tried to put pressure on the FDA to ban the cyclamate by appearing on television to drum up public support. The study initiated a crisis in Ottawa as well as in Washington. The media wanted to know what our Directorate

---

[8] Embryo and fetus are terms that refer to early and later stages of development in the womb and are used interchangeably.

159

was doing and accused health authorities of not being sensitive to public health issues.

The FDA held a meeting in Washington and invited me to evaluate Dr. Verrett's findings. I, along with other scientists, rebutted the issue, stating that the chick embryo was not a suitable specie for human risk assessment (reasons given earlier). By this time, sodium cyclamate had already become a hot issue in politics, science, and the media. Not only was the sweetener itself on trial, but so was its breakdown product, cyclohexylamine.

It soon became apparent that cyclohexylamine produced from cyclamate was the culprit for any biological effects attributed to the sweetener. Dr. McKinley, my Division Head, dropped by my lab, which was a cubbyhole with a small counter on either side of my desk. He asked me to initiate a reproduction study in rats with cyclohexylamine and to collaborate with other researchers in the Directorate who were already involved in the project. He was pleased with my willingness and gave me a new technician.

In our studies (Stoltz *et al*, 1970; Khera and Stoltz, 1970; Khera *et al*, 1971) and later in others, the only clear effect observed was on male fertility in rats, and at very high doses, which did not justify an outright ban of the sweetener. The FDA had already banned the sweetener in the U.S. Our Directorate, justifiably, continued to allow the sale of cyclamate as a tabletop sweetener, but stopped its widespread application in popular soft drinks. Ottawa, relying on its own scientific assessment, parted company with Washington.

On the heels of cyclamate came another crisis. In 1969, Dr. John W. Olney, a psychiatrist at Washington University, published in *Science* that MSG (monosodium glutamate) caused irreversible damage to infant mice when injected *intraperitoneally* (a narrow cavity enclosed by the abdominal wall). MSG is a sodium salt of glutamic acid, an amino acid, that occurs naturally in humans and is still sold under the name "Accent." It is widely used as a flavor enhancer in many foods. Dr. McKinley asked me to conduct reproduction studies on MSG, which I started immediately.

My studies, as many others, were done by oral dosing of MSG – a route of choice in humans. They failed to show any adverse effects on the fetus or newborn. Dr. Olney's positive results had come as a consequence of injecting the MSG. MSG was banned from use in baby foods because it served no useful purpose. But, its use in adult food remained unchanged. An important lesson from the MSG saga was that the route of exposure in animal tests should simulate that in humans. This is just one example that demonstrates how the principles of our testing technology, now the mainstay of safety assessment, evolved.

In the wake of the controversies that surrounded cyclamate and MSG, scientists from our Directorate developed closer working ties with FDA scientists exchanging information, opinions, and decisions before they were made public. We discussed important issues over the phone or when attending annual meetings of the Society of Toxicology.

Some important questions remained, though. What criteria separate a good and an acceptable study from a bad one? In evaluating human safety, do minor variations in development carry a weight equal to that of major malformations? Do chemicals have an exposure level that can be considered safe for humans? I was sensitive to this gap in knowledge, and I devoted my future research to clarifying some of these issues.

The safety issue of cyclamate and MSG brought the new science of Teratology to the forefront. The next two decades, 1970s and 1980s, would become significant in the history of this science when both the FDA and our Directorate were held under siege by a succession of crises ignited by Agent Orange, methylmercury, red dye Amaranth, blighted potatoes, caffeine, PCBs, and scabby wheat. Regulators and scientists in both organizations worked in tandem to provide insight and knowledge in the development of a universal safety system, in which Canada played a key role.

The Devastation of Agent Orange

Agent Orange was the name given to the herbicide 2,4,5-T and 2,4-D mixed equally in 55-gallon containers that were painted with orange color-coded stripes (T – trichlorophenoxyacetic acid, D – dichlorophenoxyacetic acid). These and other herbicides had been in use since the 1950s, well before the law required testing for human safety. They were extensively applied to crops, rangeland, timber, and utility right-of-way for brush control.

In 1966, Agent Orange and other defoliants were sprayed over two-thirds of South Vietnam to deny cover, refuge, and food to the Viet Cong in a concentration about 13 times higher than what was used in Canada and the U.S. All vegetation, birds, and insects died after spraying, and within three months the jungle was as silent as a graveyard. Cows and pigs fed on sprayed food became sick and died. By October 31, 1971, 10.5 to 12 million gallons of Agent Orange and Agent Purple (a mixture containing 1,4-D) had been sprayed on Southeast Asia's five million acres of jungle and cropland, an area about the size of Connecticut (Linedecker, 1982). The soldiers who were spraying did not wear masks or protective clothing.

In 1966-67, the North Vietnamese press, Saigon papers, and Catholic representatives of the National Liberation Front claimed the defoliant was causing epidemics of miscarriages and deformed babies. The news was disseminated worldwide, attracting the attention of the American Congress in 1969. In October of that year, the spraying program in Vietnam was reduced by 25 percent, but the data on which this decision was based was not released until December. Meanwhile, the media had already damned, not only 2,4,5-T, but all phenoxy herbicides (Clegg and Khera, 1973).

The FDA commissioned Bionetic Research Laboratories to conduct teratology studies on 2,4,5T. Their studies showed that the compound was "teratogenic" in mice and rats. Before the data was published (Courtney *et al*, 1970), the FDA sent a pre-publication copy to our Director, Dr. McKinley. Dow Chemical Corporation, the major producer of 2,4,5-T had analyzed the compound before the publication appeared and found that the samples used in the published Bionetic study contained 27 ppm of an impurity generated during the manufacturing process. The impurity was 2,3,7,8-tetrachlorodibenzo-*para*-dioxin. Based on additional information that they had, authorities at Dow believed that the dioxin and not 2,4,5-T was responsible for the teratogenic effects reported by Bionetic.

The FDA Director, authorities at Dow, and Dr. McKinley discussed the possibility of doing a joint project to investigate the effects of the above chemicals on the fetus. They agreed on an experimental protocol, and I subsequently met with a representative of Dow in Ottawa. He offered to provide all three laboratories with the required samples of 2,4,5-T (without impurities) and 2,4-D. The three laboratories then, individually, would investigate the 2,4,5-T and 2,4-D samples, and also chlorodioxin (the impurity), which was purified and provided by Dr. A.E. Pohland of FDA. The purpose was to determine whether certain variables, such as the investigator, fetal evaluation method, and other conditions in the three laboratories would influence the results.

Upon completion of the work, I presented the results on March 8, 1971 at the 10th Annual Meeting of the Society of Toxicology in Washington. My studies showed that the two phenoxy acids were teratogenic in rats, but at high doses (Khera and McKinley, 1972). An FDA official invited me to present the results again two days later at a specially arranged meeting attended by the U.S. Surgeon General and FDA authorities.

In September 1973, the American Chemical Society arranged a symposium on "Chlorodioxin – Origin and Fate" at its semi-annual meeting in Washington where all three laboratories presented their results, which were all similar to ours. In my study, 2,3,7,8-tetrachlorodibenzo-*para*-dioxin caused major malformations at a daily dose of 0.25 µg/kg (four thousandth of one mg) (Khera and Ruddick, 1973). It was the most toxic chemical I have ever worked with.

Compared to their use in Vietnam, spraying of the two defoliants on Canadian and U.S. soil was more selective, far less frequent, and at lower concentrations. Canada had not participated in the Vietnam war and consequently had no war veterans. Nevertheless, emotions ran high. The manufacturing process was modified so that 2,4,5-T had negligible levels of 2,3,7,8-TCDD (which was never present in 2,4-D). This offered the defoliant a reprieve. Its safety, however, remained a hotly debated issue throughout the 1970s. The defoliants were linked to sarcoma, non-Hodgkin's lymphoma, and Hodgkin's disease in war veterans, appearing several years after their return. A national Vietnam Task Force on Agent Orange was formed to unite veteran groups, scientists, lawyers, and church organizations. A court case failed to establish that 2,4,5-T was a risk to human health. It became clear that people with legal backgrounds could interpret data differently. If proof of a chemical's risk to human health is not validated by science, how can it be validated by law?

On February 28, 1979, the use of 2,4,5-T was suspended when it was linked to miscarriages in women in Alsea, Oregon. It was later banned. In 2003, the U.S. Institute of Medicine linked Agent Orange with lymphocytic leukemia in war veterans.

In 1973, I was invited to attend the American Association of Laboratory Animal Science's 24th Annual Session, held October 1-5 in Miami Beach, to give a seminar on "Selection of laboratory animals for predicting hazards of reproductive organ Teratogenesis." Dr. McGowan, head of our animal colony, also attended the meeting. (He later became Assistant Deputy Minister of Agriculture Canada.) He was always very cooperative and accommodating. We got along well and traveled together to Miami Beach where we shared a suite. One evening before dinner, we were sipping beer in our room, looking out at the beach. Dr. McGowan asked me out of the blue,

"How did you get to where you are? How did you make it in our country? I mean, you are already famous. You are one of 40 scientists in our building, yet your animals occupy 17 percent of the space in my colony!" I was taken aback by his questions since I had not assessed myself as a scientist. I answered, thinking aloud, that it was probably because I moved into a new science in which both my Directorate and I were equally interested. I was the right person, at the right place, at the right time.

Methylmercury in Fish

For years, several pulp and paper mills and chlorealkali plants in Canada had been spewing out tens of thousands of pounds of mercury-laced industrial waste into the waterways of Quebec, Manitoba, and Ontario. The Wabigoon-English-Winnipeg river system was so polluted from the Dryden Chemical Company's waste that mercury levels in its fish ranged from 10-28 parts per million (ppm) (Bligh, 1970; Fimreite and Reynolds, 1973) and were the highest in the western hemisphere. Fish from Clay Lake had 10-17 ppm.

The Ojibwa and Walpole Indians living on the waterway of the White Dog, Grassi Narrows, and Kenora reserves were at great risk because fish was an important part of their diet. Methylmercury pollution in the United States was not any different; 38 of its chloralkali plants were discharging industrial waste, polluting lakes and waters in 33 of its states (D'Itri and D'Itri, 1977).

At the end of 1969, a lot of public attention was focused on Canadian waterways when the federal Department of Fisheries and Forestry temporarily suspended commercial fishing from Winnipeg and Cedar Lakes and the Saskatchewan and Red Rivers. The government set a temporary action level of 0.5 ppm in fish. Any fish containing higher levels was banned from human consumption. Soon afterwards, the United States followed suit, instituting the same action level. In both countries, the maximum allowable daily intake of 0.03 mg of mercury was comparable to the weekly provisional tolerance intake of 0.2 mg/person subsequently proposed in the Sixteenth Report by FAO/WHO in 1972. Simply put, a person could eat in a week, 14 ounces of fish fillet containing 0.5 ppm (1 g = 0.035 oz), an arbitrary weekly intake that needed to be validated.

The ban on fish containing more than 0.5 ppm of mercury not only raised health issues for Canadian aboriginals residing on contaminated lakes, but also had devastating economic effects on the fishery and tourism industries.

Tourists going to fly-in fishing camps or those visiting Canadian waterways for recreational fishing disappeared.

Human poisoning with methylmercury had been observed in two large scale outbreaks. The first was in 1953 in Japan's Minamata Bay (Takeushi, 1972; Doi and Hi, 1975) where people consumed fish that had appeared healthy but had up to 5 ppm of methylmercury (Irukayama, 1968; Kitamura, 1968). These fish came from waterways that only contained 0.01 ppm of methylmercury. The second was in Iraq (1971-72) where 450 of the 6,580 patients hospitalized died from eating bread that had been made from wheat treated with mercurial fungicide.

The Japanese and Iraqi studies showed that the fetus was at least four times more sensitive to methylmercury poisoning than adults and had 20-30 percent more mercury than the mother. Mercury had been passed on to the infant through the mother's milk, rendering them more susceptible (Harada, 1968; Murakami, 1972). Some mothers gave birth to apparently healthy babies who later developed symptoms and died. The condition was characterized by infantile cerebral palsy, overall retardation in development, undersized brain, mental deficiency, tunnel vision, and a lateral squint of the eye. This poisoning was called "Congenital or Fetal Minamata Disease."

Minamata epidemics had shown that the cat was one of the most sensitive species to methylmercury poisoning (Harada, 1968) and quite possibly the most suitable species to evaluate its safety in humans.

In 1970, the Directorate gave me a laboratory that was about five times bigger than my previous one. I was busy designing and conducting experiments on cyclohexylamine, 2,4,5-T, 2,4-D, TCDD, and MSG with a large number of animals on various tests. As the work increased, so did the number of my technicians, until I had five, compared to the one or two that a scientist in our building was entitled to. As always during my entire career, I did most of the literature review and writing at home on weekends and annual vacations. In the laboratory, I personally reviewed the daily observations made by my technicians and verified any that seemed unusual. I firmly believed that, as a scientist, I was solely responsible for the accuracy of my results.

One day, while standing in line at the bank to cash my paycheck, I felt a tap on my shoulder. I turned around, and there was Dr. McKinley with his usual smile. He said, "Kun, we have a problem. We have to do some work on methylmercury to establish tolerance levels in fish from secure data." I replied, "All right, I'd be happy to do it, provided..." He intercepted saying, "Yeah, yeah, I know, you need another technician." He then asked me to drop by his office that afternoon for further discussions.

Toward the end of 1971, the Medical Research Council of Canada granted a one-year fellowship to Dr. Sonia A. Tabacova of Bulgaria tenable at the Food and Drug Directorate with Dr. McKinley. She had chosen to work in teratology and was assigned to my laboratory. Now, we were eight, and my laboratory was abuzz with activity.

I immediately began conducting experimental studies with mice and rats (dosed daily with methylmercury by oral route, sometimes mixed in food) to assess the effects on some phases of their reproduction (Khera, 1973; Khera and Tabacova, 1973). The highest daily dose that showed no effect on any aspect of reproduction was 0.1 mg/body weight/kg. Up to that time, cats were thought to be more appropriate but had never been systematically used in teratology studies because they come in heat only twice a year; knowing the precise onset of pregnancy was not always possible. I developed a methodology to induce oestrus in cats at will and mate them with tomcats held in captivity. Cats with pregnancies timed in this way were dosed daily with four graded doses of methylmercury during most of their gestation period. An additional non-treated group served as a control.

Our studies demonstrated that symptoms of methylmercury poisoning, mercury levels in the blood and brain of the fetus and their mothers, brain damage at microscopic levels, and many other features of poisoning found in the cats were similar to those reported in humans. Of all the endpoints that were investigated, the one found most sensitive was brain damage at microscopic level. The no-effect daily dose was 0.03 mg of mercury/kg/body weight (Khera, 1973b; Khera et al, 1974), 60 times lower than the FAO/WHO provisional tolerance intake enforced by the Canadian-U.S. governments. The decreed tolerance level was now backed up by firm data in a specie that reacted to methylmercury the same as human beings.

Subsequently, I extended the cat studies to include eight more chemicals with known fetal effects in humans (including thalidomide). These chemicals served as reference standards. The responses to these in the cat were comparable to those reported in humans (Khera, 1975, 1976; Khera et al, 1976b; Khera and Iverson, 1978; Khera, 1979, 1979b). The use of the cat in teratology studies was thus validated, and since then, the specie has been used for similar studies.

The much feared outbreak of mercury poisoning in Canada and the U.S. never happened. Two Canadian aboriginals, both tourist guides for recreational fishing, died of undetermined causes. Two more cases were reported in the United States, but both recovered after changing their diet. One had suffered from insomnia and anxiety and the other from numbness in the fingertips and trouble focusing the eyes (D'Itri and D'Itri, 1977). I am not aware of any other cases. However, the controversy on how much fish contaminated with methylmercury a pregnant woman can eat is far from over.

Interestingly, mercury contamination showed up in unlikely places – waterways at the northern tip of British Columbia and in "museum specimens of seven tuna caught 52 and 93 years ago and a swordfish taken 25 years ago tested at levels equivalent with contemporary specimens" (Miller *et al*, 1972). Apparently, we had been consuming mercury in marine fish with no known toxic effects for a long time. A positive result that came out of the mercury crisis was a ministerial prohibition against dumping mercury contaminated affluence in waterways.

Red Food Color

Amaranth, known in the U.S. as FD&C (food, drug, and coloring) Red No. 2, has been used virtually in all foods colored red since the turn of the 20th century. In 1970, a Russian study (Shtenberg and Gavrilenko, 1970) linked it to birth defects and stillbirths in rats. The Directorate provided me with a translation of the Russian study for evaluation. The study failed to reach research standards, but I thought that it would be foolhardy to ignore the results. I set out to determine if the results were reproducible.

In January 1972, the FDA cut back on the use of amaranth in foods after its own study (Collins *et al*, 1972) associated it with the death of embryos in rats. Meanwhile, a study by Dr. Kaplinger and collaborators under contract from the color industry was ready for publication. A crisis had been brewing in Washington between the FDA hierarchy and attorneys of the color industry on whether or not to ban the use of amaranth in food. The FDA was advised to look at the data in Kaplinger's and my studies before making a final decision.

An ad hoc advisory committee on Red No. 2 was set up by the FDA to hold a meeting on June 6, 1974. An FDA official (I cannot remember her name) invited me and Dr. Kaplinger to present our findings. Upon arrival at the FDA building's reception, I wrote my name on an attendance sheet and was given an agenda for the meeting. The receptionist had failed to tell me that I was to sit in a designated seat in the front row along with the other speakers, so I sat down in the last row. I scanned the agenda and, seeing that I was the opening speaker, started arranging my slides for projection. Just before the meeting started, the FDA official found me and introduced herself. She asked me to move to my designated seat saying, "I'm sorry; I couldn't recognize you since you do not look like a Canadian." I spontaneously quipped, "What does a Canadian look like?" An embarrassed smile was her answer.

Canadians then were often perceived as British, though the definition of Canadian had already started to become more complicated with the large number of immigrants from Asia, North Africa, and the West Indies. In science, the nationality of a scientist does not matter, since science has global perspective and serves the world. At least, that was what I thought.

Dr. Kaplinger and I made our presentations, and in the discussions that followed, our studies were judged to be well executed and valid in repudiating doubts that had emerged on the use of amaranth. Our studies were pivotal in the FDA's decision to restore amaranth in foods at its previous level. Both studies were published (Kaplinger *et al*, 1974; Khera *et al*, 1974).

Three years after the problem of fetal safety of amaranth ingestion appeared to have been resolved, a reproduction study in cats, a specie not previously used in amaranth investigations, renewed doubts on its safety (FDA, 1975). The study had serious shortcomings, among them the fact that it was done on a small number of pregnant cats. However, the Bureau of Veterinary Products regulating the safety of pet foods thought it was good enough and banned its use in cat food. This made its use in human food uncertain. I had a cat colony and also the methodology; therefore, Dr. McKinley asked me to do an investigation. I met with Duke to get his comments on a draft experimental protocol that contained all the details of the project. After the meeting, he decided it was time to have my laboratory accredited. In those days, there was no national or international scientific committee that officially accredited a toxicology or teratology laboratory. A visit by a group of highly reputed scientists and their joint voice of agreement was enough for a fledgling laboratory to be recognized. A laboratory had to be headed by a qualified scientist producing first rate research, be well-equipped, and appended to an appropriate animal housing facility.

Duke invited about 15 scientists and bureaucrats from the FDA, the color industry, as well as Dr. Joseph Borzelleca, the Secretary of the Society of Toxicology. They all converged in Ottawa at the appointed time. I presented my experimental plan, they offered their comments, and a discussion followed. I took them to the animal colony, which had about 120 cats ready for the investigation. Some of them joked that I had the biggest "cat house" in North America. They were affable and impressed. At the end of the day, my laboratory had been accredited for teratology studies by my peer group. It had taken me a little over 11 years to get recognition in a new country and in a new science.

The study was completed and published (Khera *et al*, 1976). It showed no adverse effects on any aspect of fetal development. At last, the issue of the safety of amaranth on reproduction had been laid to rest.

The Safety of Caffeine

The safety of caffeine became a hotly debated issue in 1979-80. Coffee and tea had been a part of the human diet since time immemorial. However, more pregnant women were drinking large quantities of coffee, and this was raising concerns on its safety. Studies in animals had failed to resolve the issue since adverse fetal effects in some studies were countered by their absence in others. This disagreement appeared primarily to be due to the difference in administering the caffeine to pregnant rats. When it was administered at high doses once daily (single bolus) by oral route, it gave positive results; whereas, when it was made available *ad libertum* in a solution of drinking water, it had no effect. There was also a difference in the interpretation of caffeine-related retarded growth of the sternum (breastbone).

Dr. Tom Collins and his FDA co-workers had completed a well-controlled and detail-oriented study in rats with caffeine administered as a single daily bolus. They submitted it to Dr. Colby, Jr., the Director of the FDA, who invited Dr. Carol Kimmel of the EPA and myself to jointly assess the study and interpret the results. Carol and I both agreed that the study was well executed and that retarded development of the sternum was its major finding. Retarded development of the sternum had been one of the most common observations in teratology investigations and was always a subject of controversial interpretation. We stated that, in our opinion, it could hardly be considered a malformation, since it occurred in association with reduced fetal weight and would disappear soon after birth after catching up in body weight.

The FDA study was later published (Collins *et al*, 1983).

Our Director of Research insisted that I conduct a study in rats on caffeine in drinking water. I did and got essentially negative results. I decided not to publish a negative study. There were enough out there already. In addition to caffeine-related retarded development of the sternum, several other chemicals were causing similar minor structural changes and had teratologists baffled as to their significance. It was doubtful whether or not these chemicals should be classified teratogenic. The International Life Sciences Institute in Washington invited me give a talk on fetal aberrations at their Third International Workshop on Caffeine in Hunt Valley, Baltimore. This prompted me to review the literature. This review, along with my own laboratory experience, helped me develop a paper in which I described a number of specific minor changes or fetal aberrations. These were either transitory or permanent, but invariably innocuous to the incumbent. I also offered suggestions on whether potential offending chemicals should be classified as teratogenic or not. The paper was later published (Khera, 1981) and became a popular source of reference.

Vomitoxin (scabby wheat)

Vomitoxin, or DON (4-deoxynivalenol) is produced by the *Fusarium* mold which causes fungal disease in wheat known as scabby wheat. It appears in the form of red kernels. The mold grows and forms vomitoxin and is found on other cereal grains such as corn and oats. The toxin causes adverse effects in laboratory animals and is suspected of inducing toxicity in humans and animals.

A method to detect vomitoxin became available for the first time in 1980, and the first crop to be analyzed was the 1980 winter wheat harvested in eastern Canada. The scientist was a colleague of mine (Scott, 1980). The concentrations of vomitoxin in Ontario wheat ranged from 0.01 to 4.3 ppm, and in Quebec they were worse. In 1981, the harvested crop in Quebec contained such high levels of vomitoxin (up to 5 ppm) that it was not recommended for human consumption (Scott, 1981). Large surveys conducted in 1981 and 1982 revealed that vomitoxin contamination, quite high at times, was widespread throughout Canada and the U.S. (Romer, 1983). After that, contamination has commonly been found in North America (House, 1991), posing health hazards to humans and causing continued economic losses to wheat farmers. The frequent presence of mold mycotoxin was not a sufficient reason to condemn wheat for human use.

In 1981, the federal government of Canada commissioned our Food Directorate to conduct animal studies on vomitoxin to elucidate its health effects. As part of the program, I was asked to do reproduction and teratology studies to assess its risks in order to set legal tolerance levels of vomitoxin in wheat. The Directorate needed immediate toxicity data to set these levels, but had very small quantities of purified vomitoxin for the required tests. I was asked to come up with a study as quickly as possible. I conducted a preliminary study in mice, which was completed within eight weeks (Khera, 1982). It was this study, I presume, that formed the basis of the provisional tolerance levels of 0.1 ppm in wheat flour for bread, and 0.3 ppm for wheat flour used in cakes and biscuits. To meet these levels, the cereal-making industry had to reject large shipments of wheat, raising the ire of wheat farmers in eastern Canada.

I followed up on the above study with an investigation in rats and another in mice (Khera *et al*, 1984) and rabbits (Khera *et al*, 1986). As a result of these and other studies from our Directorate, tolerance levels of vomitoxin were increased to 1 ppm in bread flour and 2 ppm for wheat flour used for cakes and biscuits. This data was also used by both the U.S. and England.

Ethylenethiourea (fungicide)

Ethylenethiourea (ETU) was a model or exemplary compound which I used to understand the development of hydrocephalus, an abnormal accumulation of fluid in the brain of a fetus or newborn that enlarges the head and causes mental deficiency. ETU is a common breakdown product of several fungicides that belonged to the ethylene-bis-dithiocarbamate group of chemicals which are sprayed on a wide variety of vegetables. These fungicides have now been banned.

In rats, ETU had no effect on a pup when administered after it was born, but caused a highly selective killing of neurons or brain cells in the fetus that culminated in congenital hydrocephalus. The selective killing was observed only during the last ten days of fetal development. ETU was, therefore, highly selective in attacking only the early stages of brain development. ETU gave me an insight on some of the phenomena that are basic to teratology. It captivated my attention for 17 years with results reported in 16 papers (see Bibliography).

Pesticidal Formulations

A search of published and unpublished data (stored in our Directorate) revealed that a large number of pesticides appeared to have never been tested for fetal effects. These pesticides had been in use long before the requirements for teratology data were enacted. I initiated a research program to fill this gap.

A pesticide is sold as a formulation that contains the active pesticide itself, chemicals to hold the pesticide in suspension, and synergists or chemicals that enhance its intended lethal effects. Over a number of years, I investigated purified pesticides or synergists either alone or as a formulation sold on the market.[9]

My Contribution to Testing Guidelines

As I pointed out before, during the period from May 1960 to the early 1970s, the number of teratogenic chemicals and the number of teratology investigations grew rapidly. A number of these studies reported insufficient or unconvincing data that raised unsubstantiated doubts on the safety of many chemicals. Human beings had been using a lot of these chemicals for decades without any apparent ill effect. Food additives, such as amaranth, benzoic acid, carrageen, MSG, and drugs such as aspirin and cold medicines are just a few examples. Regulatory agencies in several countries were wary of these faulty studies, since they were faced with the dilemma of either allowing a useful chemical to stay in use and face bad publicity or ban one on invalid grounds and face the manufacturer in a court of law.

A shortage of suitable data, the common thread in many of these studies, was due to inappropriate design and conduct. Dr. Goldenthal of the FDA had rectified some of these deficiencies by proposing guidelines to determine the safety of pharmaceutical drugs (1966) for commercial use, but most researchers outside pharmaceutical circles remained unaware.

Guidelines provide a scientist with detailed systematic information on

---

[9] These included Hexachlorobenzene, Diquat, Paraquat, Halogenated Benzenes, Mirex (fire ant killer), Photomirex, Linuron, Malathion, Methoxychlor, Piperonyl Butoxide, Biphenyl, Phasolone, Dimethoate, Diuron, Lindane (ant killer), Maleic, Hydrazide, Daminozide, Ethoxyquin, Thiabendazole (also used to treat pinworms in humans), Naled, Pyrethrum, and Rotenone (common garden pesticide).

how to plan and execute tests, collect information, analyze data, and interpret results. They are based on published data and personal wisdom derived from reasoning and experience. Writing guidelines is like putting together a jigsaw puzzle that comes with some of its interlocking pieces missing. A puzzle solver has to furnish the appropriately shaped pieces to complete the puzzle. Thus, guidelines also point out what is known and what is assumed and needs future research. As the facts increase, the contribution of objective wisdom decreases. Guidelines, therefore, need to be updated from time to time.

In 1973, the Health Protection Branch in Canada formed working groups, of which I was a member, to develop testing guidelines. Over a period of about three months, we met to define the type of tests required for human safety from animal studies. It was not a cookbook recipe, but was quite comprehensive. We then compiled all the information in a book entitled "Document: Carcinogenesis, Mutagenesis, Teratogenesis." It was called the "Red Book" after the color of its cover. In order to ensure wide distribution, it was made available free of charge. The then USSR requested 50 copies for its research institutes. The first printing evaporated in no time.

While at a meeting in 1977, I was approached by a scientist from the U.S. National Academy of Sciences in Washington. He asked me to become a member of the Subcommittee on Reproduction and Teratogenesis. Our mandate was to develop a revised set of guidelines that would reflect the state-of-the-art, determine how tests should be done, and, more importantly, what areas needed further research. The published guidelines were entitled "Principles and procedures for evaluating the toxicity of household substances" (Harbison *et al*, 1977).

Developing countries did not have the expertise to design their own guidelines, so officials at the World Health Organization's International Programme on Chemical Safety decided to produce guidelines that would be acceptable to all the countries of the world. In 1982, I was approached by Dr. Michel Mercier of WHO, who asked me to be the "Rapporteur" of the group. The group was comprised of a large number of scientists from all over the world, including countries from the "Iron Curtain." During 1983-84, the entire group met for extensive discussions three times, in St. Petersburg (Russia), Prague (Czechoslovakia), and Geneva (Switzerland), and the core group met three more times in Geneva. As Rapporteur, I incorporated all views, wrote chapters, and edited the guidelines (WHO, 1984).

By then, many countries and even their different agencies had their own guidelines with many variations in data requirement. Once more, I was invited to put together a working group to produce guidelines for human safety assessment, this time by the International Life Sciences Institute in Washington, D.C. Duke and D.J. Clegg were my collaborators (Khera *et al*, 1989).

Chapter 18: The Peak of My Career

Maternal Toxicity

The history of birth defects dates back to 6500 BC and has been well documented (see Warkany, 1971). Out of curiosity, Aristotle was known to have produced grossly malformed chickens by injecting eggs with substances such as sand. The record of birth defects is one of the richest among sciences and includes the malformed or deformed people seen in side shows, circuses, carnivals, and country fairs, in addition to the myths, gods (elephant-headed Ganesh, ten-headed Ravanna for example), mermaids, and Siamese twins that inspire love, fear, and awe.

Until the mid-1980s, there was a widely held view in the scientific community that following exposure to chemicals during pregnancy, all a mother did was channel the chemical through the placenta to the embryo or fetus and break it down to its end products for excretion. The chemicals or their end products produced their toxic effects by hitting the fetus directly.

One of the most important struggles of my professional life took place in the ten years before my retirement when I strove to convince my peers that this view was inaccurate. My research provided clear evidence that a vast majority of chemicals, when given at high doses during pregnancy, could also affect the fetus indirectly; that is, they first caused toxic effects in the mother or placenta, which in turn caused toxic effects on the fetus. The research on toxic effects in the mother created a new field which then modified the method used to interpret animal data for human safety. Investigations on how chemicals or drugs induced congenital defects shifted their emphasis from the embryo per se to the mother-placenta-embryo axis. My contribution to this field and these changes was a major achievement of my career.

Toxic effects of chemicals manifest themselves differently in the embryo than in pregnant animals. In the embryo, these effects are called embryotoxicity and are characterized by reduced body weight, malformations or aberrations, and death. They may occur in the womb and may be observed in the newborn. In the pregnant animal, signs and symptoms of toxic effects or maternal toxicity vary greatly and consist of reduced food or water intake and a decrease in body weight, associated with marked alterations in behavior (aggressiveness or sedation), respiration, and other body functions.

By 1976, extensive data from human studies had identified about 40 chemicals, including drugs and environmental agents that caused or were suspected of causing adverse effects on fetal development following their use or exposure during pregnancy. Included in this group were the prescription drugs thalidomide, isotretinoin (vitamin A), DES (diethylstilboestrol, an anti-abortion drug), diphenylhydantoin, phenobarbital, and trimethadione (anti-seizure drugs), alcohol, heroin, and cocaine, and environmental agents such as radiation and methylmercury. In animal studies, all of the above had shown embryotoxic effects.

In striking contrast to the negative findings in human studies, animal studies had identified an additional 800 chemicals causing adverse fetal effects (Staples, 1976). In the succeeding six years, this animal to human ratio of 800 to 40 had further increased (Larsson *et al*, 1982), and I can say with confidence that this ratio continues to increase.

The then current strategy of risk assessment was based on the above information and rested on the following premise: almost all suspected or known human teratogens had demonstrated some sort of embryotoxic effects when tested in laboratory animals. Therefore, if a new chemical was hazardous to human development, it would most probably be recognized in animal reproduction studies. On the contrary, not all of the chemicals so far found embryotoxic in animals were noxious to the human fetus. And so, fetal studies in animals continued to identify many chemicals that may not have been harmful to the human fetus at all. Yet, these chemicals would not be marketed because they were regulated as harmful to humans. Why? Because it was, and is, prudent to err on the side of safety. Many scientists, myself included, believe that such a basis for arriving at safety was questionable.

I found it difficult to comprehend the difference in the animal to human ratio. There was one possibility. Experimental animals were closely observed for signs of abortion or fetal wastage, and any such occurrence could be related to the test drug. However, in pregnant women, it was impossible to assign definite causes of abortions or early miscarriages to any one chemical because of the simultaneous exposure to environmental agents, drugs, alcohol, and tobacco. Even if this possibility were accepted, the above gap in animal/human ratio could not be bridged.

I was tantalized by the enormous difference in these numbers. This drove me to do an extensive review of the literature in which I analyzed the effects of diverse chemicals on embryos, term fetuses, and their mothers. I had extensive data from which I abstracted clear statements that were testable in future investigations. The core of my conclusions was as follows:

> Maternal toxicity by itself, irrespective of the type of chemical or physical agent causing it, can produce embryotoxic effects. These effects appear in a consistent pattern in term fetuses – i.e., a gradient of the same type of malformations and aberrations. A chemical administered to a pregnant animal produces embryotoxic effects in two ways: either by acting directly on the embryo,[10] or by indirect action as a consequence of its toxic effect on the mother. I deduce that the latter type of chemical should not be labeled as teratogenic. Based on this conclusion, I propose this hypothesis on the new role of "maternal toxicity."

I presented the preliminary results of my review in June 1983 at the Teratology Society's 23rd Annual Meeting in Atlantic City. Most of my data linking embryotoxic effects to the toxic effects on the mother had come from studies on mice. Researchers who worked with other species found new reasons to look down upon the mouse as an unworthy specie to serve the human race! The vanguard of teratology rejected my hypothesis without a second thought. To them, this view was stunning and sounded heretical. The overall response of the audience was lukewarm.

Undeterred, I continued my reviews, this time concentrating on studies from rats, hamsters, and rabbits and presented the results at the Society's next Annual Meeting. The data this time was much more conclusive in support of my hypothesis. In addition to reiterating my hypothesis, I proposed a complete scrutiny of toxic effects in the mother and suggested new endpoints for future studies, since ties of toxic effects in the mother and its fetus had taken on a new meaning. (It is interesting to note that, within a few weeks of the meeting, a directive authored by an anonymous EPA official was published in the U.S. Government's Federal Register. The directive, with no reference to my work, stated that a complete examination of maternal animals was now obligatory, and it spelled out the same criteria that I had proposed at the meeting.)

---

[10] At the time, this was the widely held view among scientists.

The three reviews which I had presented at the Teratology Society meetings appeared in three separate publications. In my first paper (1984), I enunciated the hypothesis with data on mice. My second paper (1985) contained tabularly arranged detailed data from a large number of studies with reference to their published journals. At the 1986 Teratology Society meeting, a librarian caught up to me and told me that an EPA official, who wanted to ascertain the accuracy of my review, had asked her to collect photocopies of all the papers I had cited in my review. I was surprised and yet pleased that my hypothesis had penetrated the EPA, an important regulatory agency.

My hypothesis kindled passions and stirred up emotions, yet failed to provoke much action. Some scientists felt that their entire concepts were being challenged. Others thought that the teratogenicity of chemicals tested at very high doses would be shadowed by doubts that maternal toxicity was the possible underlying cause. Hardly anybody thought that teratology had sprouted a new concept worthy of further investigation.

In September 1984, the Toxicology Forum invited me to give a seminar on the predictive value of current testing methods at their European meeting in Geneva. I talked at length on maternal toxicity and had long discussions on my hypothesis with FDA regulators, including Dr. Goldenthal. The participants seemed genuinely interested.

In July 1985, again at the Teratology Society's Annual Meeting held in Callaway Gardens, Georgia, I further supported my hypothesis by presenting data from human studies in which, once again, maternal toxicity seemed closely connected to adverse effects on the fetus or newborn.

I submitted this review to *Issues and Reviews in Teratology.* It was rejected. The editor, Harold Kalter, who happened to be a friend of mine, told me that his journal did publish controversial issues, but that my hypothesis was far too outlandish to be considered. However, it was not too outlandish for *C.R.C. Reviews in Toxicology,* which published it without comment in 1987.

I realized that many scientists were having a hard time grasping my hypothesis. It was clear that toxicity in the mother was associated with embryotoxic effects in 75 percent of the test chemicals. The remaining 25 percent had produced toxic effects in the mother but not in the embryo. Obviously, maternal toxicity was occurring in two forms: one in the presence of and the other in the absence of fetal effects. The two forms could not be differentiated by external signs in the pregnant animals.

All of a sudden, maternal toxicity caught fire. It was not just in the limelight; it became *the* most important issue. In 1986, my hypothesis led to a consensus workshop on the evaluation of maternal and developmental toxicity organized by the EPA on May 12-14 in Washington, D.C., where a panel of 50 renowned teratologists from different countries were asked to present their views. They ran high in opinions, but fell short in presenting data to refute my hypothesis. No agreement was reached on whether maternal toxicity was or wasn't the cause of fetal malformations. The panel could only agree on recommendations for future research – the most significant of which was to conduct well-planned experiments to define maternal toxicity and its role in fetal malformations. The summary of the proceedings and papers presented were published in *Teratogenesis, Carcinogenesis, Mutagenesis* (1987).

Soon after, maternal toxicity was recognized as an important issue by regulatory agencies and teratology societies worldwide. There was a quantum leap of interest in knowing what maternal toxicity could produce in the fetus and how. In 1986, I received a formal invitation from Dr. Kirsten Jacobsen of H. Lundbeck Pharmaceutical on behalf of the European Teratology Society to give a seminar at their annual conference which was held in September at Ndr. Strandvej, Denmark. Claire and I traveled to Copenhagen where we were met by organizers of the conference. Their hospitality was second to none. Kirsten and her husband Erik arranged for us to stay in a bed and breakfast near their home that was owned by a delightful couple who went out of their way to make us feel at home. We were also taken on a two-day sightseeing tour of museums and castles. The most impressive was Kronborg Castle in Elsinore, the world famous backdrop of Shakespeare's *Hamlet*.

The meeting was attended by a large number of scientists from all over the world. Almost all the scientists at the meeting attended my seminar, and maternal toxicity inspired an unprecedented interest for future research. After one of the sessions, Dr. R. Padmanabhan, a teratologist from the United Arab Republic, introduced himself and told me how much he had enjoyed reading my research papers. He then said that he felt privileged to meet me. I was deeply moved. Over the three days of discussions, I made many useful contacts and memorable encounters.

Maternal toxicity had a major impact on three areas: how chemicals and drugs act to produce toxic effects on the embryo; assessment of human safety; and defining some of the technical terms used in teratology. I presume that my hypothesis influenced terminology since, soon after, I started to notice some changes. The prefix of teratology, or the science itself, and terms such as teratogen, teratogenic, and teratologic, are derived from the Greek word *teras* meaning monster. In animal studies, terms with the prefix *terat* were discarded, and all adverse effects observed in term fetuses and newborns were renamed *reproduction effects*; thus, teratology studies became *reproduction studies*; and the science of animal teratology became *reproduction toxicity*. The science of testing in animals made almost a clean break from its direct relevance or implications to human malformations. In humans, the science of congenital malformations induced by chemicals did not undergo any name change.

The drug and chemical industry was quick to note the implications of the hypothesis on safety assessment. The industry's scientists argued with the regulatory agencies that chemicals that caused fetal aberrations at doses toxic for the mother should be regulated as toxic rather than teratogenic. Control measures for toxic chemicals were much more lenient than those for teratogens.

Regulatory agencies had difficulty dealing with the new reality. They thought that the hypothesis was an assault on a system which, to date, had worked well. The regulatory response was simple. So far, it had required data on maternal effects only to ensure that the highest dose tested had some form of toxic effect on the mother. The agencies then changed their mandate. A complete appraisal of pregnant animals became obligatory, and some new endpoints were added to measure maternal health. A new submission for approval of drugs had to have a "no observed effect level" (NOEL), or "lowest observed effect level" (LOEL) from both maternal and fetal data.

Regulatory agencies asked the chemical and pharmaceutical industries for further studies in cases where maternal toxicity and embryotoxicity occurred at the same or at similar doses. These studies were to focus on providing answers to whether a chemical caused embryotoxicity as a result of its indirect action through toxic effects in the mother or its direct action on the embryo itself. The issue could only be clarified by developing new methods and innovative procedures (Khera, 1991) that might vary from chemical to chemical. There are people who think that regulatory agencies should outline procedures to delineate the role of maternal toxicity in teratology studies. My view is that these answers have to come from research in the laboratory.

Prevention of disease by understanding its causes has always been the guiding principle of medical science. However, preventing birth defects caused by chemicals is not based on such understanding. It was my dream that one day the prevention of birth defects would also be based on understanding how the normal development of a fetus goes awry.

My hypothesis was a first step toward realizing this goal. It created a whole new realm for investigation. Could I let the hypothesis go without follow-up studies? No. Hypotheses could, depending on the results, be exhilarating or heartbreaking. I had faith in my reviews and a strong instinct that I was right. My investigative strategy included analyses of: maternal blood, a lifeline that rallies mother-placenta-embryo into an axis; the placenta and its early stages of development – the site where the exchange between the mother's blood and fetal blood takes place.

I was entering an unfamiliar area of work for which I had to acquire new knowledge, innovative techniques, and imaginative work plans. I gave myself a refresher course in the biochemistry of blood and development of the placenta. This consumed much of my free time at home for a year as well as two annual vacations. In 1987, I prepared a research proposal which I submitted to the U.S. March of Dimes for funding, since I knew they were generous in granting research money into birth defects. However, in my case, the agency refused. I then presented it to my Directorate. The proposal was accepted, and the purchase of equipment was staggered over three budget years. At last, I got started.

My investigations revealed a close association of embryotoxicity with the following five conditions of maternal health. The first four involved maternal blood, and the fifth, the placenta. (1) Disturbed concentrations of electrolytes or salt ions which, in turn, disturbed the normal movement of fluids through body tissues. (2) Blood too acidic; normal blood is slightly on the alkaline side of neutral. (3) Abnormally high levels of carbon dioxide; some chemicals speeded up a body's metabolism and carbon dioxide was the end product of this metabolism. (4) Low hemoglobin (red oxygen-carrying protein) in red blood cells or fewer red blood cells. Hemoglobin gives a piggy-back ride to vital oxygen through body tissues and to the waste carbon dioxide which the lungs exhale. (5) Marked degenerative changes in the placenta that resulted in a reduced rate of exchange between maternal blood and fetal blood.

I presented the results at different meetings between 1989 and 1991 and published them in 1991-93. The study that I published in 1991 was, I think, the best of my work. The validity of my hypothesis was subsequently confirmed by many others in different experiments (for example, Ban et al, 1989; Ozawa *et al*, 1990; Desesso and Goeringer, 1990; Sullivan Jones *et al*, 1992; Beck and Mark, 1992; Foley *et al*, 1993; Daston *et al*, 1994; Duffy *et al*, 1997; Colomina *et al*, 1998; Maurissen *et al*, 2000; Wise *et al*, 2000; Sharova *et al*, 2000; Collins *et al*, 1998).

Evaluating My Research

When an article is published in a scientific journal, the author provides references to other papers (often listed as bibliography or references cited) that are relevant to its subject matter. These references are then collected from thousands of scholarly journals, catalogued, and periodically printed by ISI (International Science Institute). They are also available on the internet from the Science Citation Index. Each cited reference is indexed so that a search shows the total number of times an author's published work has been cited, with the name, date of the publication, etc.

Depending upon the significance of the findings, an author may be cited many times, less frequently or not at all, thus providing an assessment of the scientific quality of an article and, in turn, of the scientist. During my career, I published 104 research and review papers (see bibliography). Out of curiosity, at the end of February 2002, I did a search for citations of my papers which were published between 1958, the date of my first publication, and 1993. I had been cited in 2,029 scientific articles, and five of my papers were cited over 100 times; two of them were on maternal toxicity.

The Societies

For scientists, membership in a society is essential. It facilitates professional development, meeting peer groups, and developing personal relations with other scientists. The annual general meetings provide a forum for discussions, presentation of papers on ongoing research, and study sessions. A society quite often has a journal in which its members publish the results of their research. I was a member of two societies – the Society of Toxicology and Applied Pharmacology and the Teratology Society. They differed from each other in many ways.

The Society of Toxicology

The Society of Toxicology was officially recognized in 1961 and began publishing its official journal, *Toxicology and Applied Pharmacology,* at about the same time. The first meeting I attended was the Society's fourth annual meeting in 1965. There were no more than 40 members in attendance. The atmosphere was so cordial that, at the end of the three-day meeting, I knew almost everyone. I presented a paper in which I showed photographs of ducklings hatched from Systox-treated eggs (a pesticide). Soon after the meeting, a Mrs. Woodward said, "Your ducklings had beautiful eyes." I said, "yes," and then she, her husband, and I all laughed. She and her husband owned a toxicology laboratory that did contract work for the drug industry.

I attended all the annual meetings until 1980 and then only infrequently, as the Directorate's budget was cut. The 1990 annual meeting would be my last. By then, the Society had more than 3,000 members and another journal, *Fundamental and Applied Toxicology* (first issued in 1980 in response to an increasing number of manuscripts). The type of research reported in the two journals met high standards. The members exuded warmth; the officers were good natured; and the atmosphere of the meetings was friendly and conducive to research. I always looked forward to attending the meetings. I served the society as a member of the Technical Committee for one year, the Program Committee for three years, and was Associate Editor of the *Journal of Toxicology and Applied Pharmacology* for ten years.

In 1988, the Society honored me by selecting me for the Arnold J. Lehmann Award "in recognition of scientific excellence and continuing contributions to the field of toxicology." Claire and I flew to Dallas for the award ceremony and banquet, which was held at the society's annual meeting. I was deeply touched by the president's speech, which covered the highlights of my research career. The details were published in *Toxicology and Applied Pharmacology* (see photo, p. 205).

The Teratology Society

The Teratology Society was founded in 1960, and I became a chartered member in 1967. The society's official journal was *Teratology.* Over some 25 years, I presented a large number of my papers at its annual meetings. These were subsequently published in the Society's journal. The Society had a relatively small membership, and yet, for unknown reasons, I never felt the fellowship that was extended to me in the Society of Toxicology.

One incident in particular stands out in my mind. It happened in 1976 at the annual meeting in Carmel, California. I presented a paper on offspring from rats that had been treated during pregnancy with Ethylenethiourea (a breakdown product of fungicides). The offspring could not walk normally. Instead, they hopped somewhat like the gait of a kangaroo. I showed a video starring these "hoppers" which created a dramatic effect on the audience. This congenital defect was unique and had never been reported.

Immediately after the video ended, a member of the society jumped to his feet and made a long comment. To my dismay, he proceeded to announce that this defect was not new to him. In fact, he claimed to have observed the same type of hopping with another chemical long before I did. He ended by saying that he never got around to presenting or publishing his results. In the heat of the moment, he had succeeded in deflecting much of the audience's attention onto him. I found it ironic that his results were never presented or published. Mine were published within a year (Khera and Tryphonas, 1977). This man was a past president of the Society. This example typifies the attitude of a lot of the Society's members toward my research. Given the negative response to my hypothesis on maternal toxicity, I deduced that the Society was not open to new ideas and, therefore, not an appropriate forum for me.

The Teratology Society was made up of both American and Canadian scientists. I wondered, though, if the attitude of some of its members was racially motivated. These members were the movers and shakers of the Society. Once, I asked an American friend of mine why I was being treated that way. He replied, "You don't seem to get it, do you?" confirming that much of my problems with the Society were due to my appearance and accent.

A Man of Color

When I arrived in Ottawa In 1964, there were few immigrants of dark complexion, but by the 1970s, more could be seen on the streets of downtown and in large shopping malls. As their numbers increased, so did racial prejudice. It was common practice then for immigrants with dark skins to be refused accommodation and jobs that involved dealing with the public. Employers gave strange excuses to camouflage their racial preferences. Bearded Sikhs were often confused with hippies. When a colleague of mine (Dr. Harpal S. Buttar) appeared as a candidate for work at the Drug Directorate, his superior, Dr. Blake Coldwell, asked me, "Is he a hippie?"

In 1965, while I was being examined by a dentist, she called in her assistant. She asked her to look into my mouth and said, "See, his mouth is the same color as ours even though his skin is dark." That same year, while visiting the Directorate's store, the clerk told me that, when his wife had gone to a blood donor clinic, the Red Cross nurse had refused to take her blood, saying that her skin was too dark. She had been profoundly hurt. She and her husband were recent immigrants from Central Province in India and had wanted to make a contribution to their new society. I know of several other such incidences, either from my own experience or from that of my fellow immigrants. As a result, a large number of people I know who came from India disconnected themselves from civic life in Canada and formed their own cultural groups. As for myself, I didn't find these remarks hurtful or provocative, but saw them as signs of ignorance coming from depressing failures as human beings.

Multiculturalism

Multiculturalism became an official policy of the Government of Canada in 1971. It was quite a turnaround for a country whose history in race relations had not always been laudable. Canada's population growth was due mostly to immigration from countries worldwide and represents a wide social, cultural, and linguistic range.

Discussions, arguments, and wisdom gave birth to the concept of multiculturalism and cemented diverse faiths, various languages, and different cultures. This concept replaced a policy based on group supremacy, class inclusion, and socio-centricity which was by nature nationally divisive. It was endorsed by all political parties and the general population. Canada thus achieved in a unique way a national solidarity and social cohesion.

The vast majority of Canadians and visible minorities, including myself, view this cultural mosaic as an iconic symbol of fairness and equality. However, there are opponents who continue to believe that all immigrants should be assimilated to make Canada a unicultural society. They vehemently protest against cultural pluralism. Their number is not large, but is vocal enough to cause anxiety to visible minorities who must endure their disapproval *overtly* on the street, in the school yard, at security check points in airports and at border crossings, and *covertly* in job interviews, recruitments, hiring, promotions, etc. A survey across Canada by the Canadian Policy Research Network expressed that Canadians are worried that racism and discrimination are on the rise, but say at the same time that ethnic and cultural diversity has made Canada a strong nation (Maxwell, 2002).

Covert discriminatory practices in recruitment and promotions have caused a chronic underrepresentation of visible minorities in publicly funded institutions. Minorities find themselves helpless, since discrimination is hard to prove. Two legal cases of racial preference relating to promotions have been lodged – one against the National Research Council and the other against Health Canada. In both cases, the decision was in favor of the plaintiff. However, these cases did not do much for the image or policies of the two institutions.

To help eliminate the discriminations, policymakers could include, on an ad hoc basis, at least one member of a visible minority in departmental hiring and promotion committees. Appropriately qualified members would not be difficult to find since there is no shortage of talent.

In public opinion polls, Canadians have repeatedly expressed a preference for immigrants from Europe, Latin America, or Africa for instance, with the least number from Asian countries. This preference has no apparent effect on Asians already in Canada; however, its connotations are depressing and hard to deny. Is it because of our skin color, our culture, our language, and our religions? Being of Asian descent, I can't help but feel a sense of rejection every time I read these polls. I find it strange that the majority of Canadians who take pride in cultural pluralism say that differences in culture, religion, language, and complexion of immigrants living in Canada do not matter. Why then are Asians least preferred as future immigrants? With regard to these opinion polls, I have not been able to understand why they are conducted and published. What purpose do they serve other than to reinforce preexisting racial bias?

My Work Environment

My co-workers at the Directorate were always polite and treated me with respect. At staff meetings, when it was necessary, I did not hesitate to state my opinion, even if it differed from that of others. When I was asked for my view, I provided, if needed, honest, constructive criticism. However, I always kept a cheerful distance from those in authority. In all my yearly assessments, my research was rated good to excellent. I knew I was different, but I believed that my complexion conferred a distinct advantage; not only did it set me apart from others, but my face stuck far much longer in the memory of those whom I had met, even for a brief moment.

I had job-related difficulties at the Directorate twice during my career, and neither was race related. In 1974, in the course of my annual assessment, I asked for a promotion to Research Scientist 3. As one of the most productive scientists in the Directorate, I believed I deserved it. My request was denied. A few weeks later, I received a phone call from a colleague, Dr. Bernie Becker of Abbott laboratories. He asked me if I could recommend someone for a position at Midwest Research Institute in Kansas City. I told him that I, in fact, was looking for a job. He said that the Institute would get in touch with me very soon. Within three months, I had an offer of a job from Midwest paying $5,000 more than my current salary. I handed in my resignation. The Director of the Food Directorate asked to see me in his office. He wanted to know my reasons for leaving. I told him that it was because the Directorate had refused to promote me. Right away, he promised to match the salary and promote me at the next annual appraisal, which was due in a few months. Not leaving anything to chance, I asked him to put this in writing, which he did.

In 1980, when I was section head, I told my superiors that I didn't want this position since it had additional administrative duties with no additional pay. Plus, the administrative work cut down on my research. They refused to relieve me of these duties. At that time, there was an employment exchange program in California for toxicologists. I sent in my curriculum vitae and, within a week or so, was invited by Dow Chemical Company in Michigan for an interview. Soon after my return, someone at the Directorate found out that Dow was planning to hire me. I was relieved of my duties as section head and was able to pursue my research full-time.

In both instances, I really wanted to stay in Canada because I had excellent laboratory facilities, expensive equipment, and a sizable budget. I found this package attractive, and it enabled me to do quality research and stay competitive with international toxicologists. The laboratories of the Health Protection Branch (that included the Food and Drug Laboratories) were well-poised to become a prominent research Institute. Its scientists had been acclaimed by the Society of Toxicology and the American Chemical Society. I, along with many others, thought that the Health Protection Branch would soon be considered equal to Sloan-Kettering, Salk, Stanford, or Harvard, which are national research jewels for American scholars. Sadly, this never happened, not because of a lack of talent, but because of a lack of political vision in the wake of budgetary cuts, downsizing, and golden handshakes.

My Retirement

Up to 1990, a research scientist at the Health Protection Branch had been allowed travel expenses to attend meetings once a year. This policy, however, was changed, and in the spring of 1991, I was told that I could not get travel expenses to attend any meetings that year. I was also advised that, not only would I have to cover my own expenses, I would also have to take annual vacation for the duration of my absence. This announcement came as a surprise and dealt quite a blow to me.

By then, the Society of Teratology had already accepted one of my papers for presentation. According to the bylaws of the Society, once a paper was accepted, it had to be presented at the annual meeting. By chance, Dr. Narsing Agnish, a friend and teratologist with Hoffman LaRoche based in New Jersey, learned about my inability to attend the meeting from one of my colleagues. Shortly after, I received a telephone call from Narsing, inviting me to give a seminar at LaRoche immediately before the annual meeting. LaRoche paid all my expenses!

In 1991, the contamination of fish from the St. Lawrence River was getting a lot of coverage in the media. Fish samples showed the presence of a number of chemicals, such as Furans, dioxins, methylmercury, etc. The Food Directorate was planning a study in which fish, freeze-dried and powdered, would be investigated for reproductive effects in rats. I was shown the study plan in its initial phase, but was not invited for discussions on its later phases. I later found out that the Directorate was contemplating contracting it out to a private laboratory.

These two events at work signalled to me that I had become irrelevant to the needs of the Directorate. I took retirement, effective October 20, 1992, after dedicating my life to serving the Directorate for 28 years. The teratology investigations of food-borne chemicals at the Food Directorate, which had started with my arrival in 1964, ended with my departure in 1992.

Chapter 19: My Later Years

Back in India

Every Friday, I wrote to my children, sending words of encouragement and inspiration to help build their confidence. I would remind them to give their full attention to their studies, to be sure to do their assignments, and to set goals for themselves. Awtar, Jyoti, and Nickky were still young, and I felt they needed my attention and guidance. I also urged them to assume responsibility for their lives by repeatedly assuring them of an adequate supply of money for their education, for as long as they wanted to study and in any field they chose. They and Rajinder wrote often to keep me informed of their progress. I'm certain that my absence had an impact on their lives. However, had I returned to India, I would not have had the money to finance their education, nor could I have given my daughters the weddings that they had and deserved. I might also have been a very unhappy professor, which would have had a negative impact on all of them.

I remembered how Rajinder and I had bickered over money to pay for flour, lentil, and beans. We worried constantly about repaying what had been bought on credit. Some of those creditors even came pounding on our door demanding payment. Raising six children on a meager income had not been easy. Those days were hard to forget.

After Bibi's death, Rajinder moved from Hissar to Ludhiana where Jag had been admitted to the Engineering College. When, in 1966, I received a promotion with retroactive pay, I sent Rajinder all of it (equivalent to Rs20,000), thus enabling her to buy a house next to the Agricultural University.

Rajinder and I discussed the problem of finding suitable matches in Canada for our daughters. Because the Indian community in Canada and the United States combined in the 1960s was very small, we agreed that the interest of our daughters was much better served in Ludhiana, where they could finish their education, find good jobs, and, above all, be among our relatives who could help in the search for suitable matches.

Up to 1966, I had been sending money regularly to Rajinder in the form of a bank draft at a rate that gave about Rs4.6 per dollar, with minor fluctuations. This was the official rate, and it was strictly controlled by the Government of India. Deak and Company in Toronto was popular with Indians who were sending money back home, and they gave Rs6 per dollar. The difference was substantial. In a telephone conversation, a company representative explained that neither my beneficiary nor I would be doing anything unlawful. Only the Indian Branch of Deak and Company could be sued for trading dollars to rupees. He guaranteed that their transactions in India were safeguarded: the head office in Toronto sent coded messages to Branch employees in major Indian cities; an employee would then travel to the beneficiary's residence to deliver the cash. Thus assured, I started sending money through Deak and Company. After about a year, Deak's Branch in India switched from delivery by hand to bank draft by mail. The Government of India intercepted one of the bank drafts and the Reserve Bank of India was soon hounding Rajinder with letters. Awtar sent me photocopies of them relating their dilemma. The bank had charged Rajinder with receiving money by illegal means and gave her a choice to either fight it in court or pay a fine of Rs3,000. She accepted the latter, and I paid the fine.

This incident frightened me and deterred me from visiting India. If I went, I thought I might have to go through a long, dragged out civil suit which could jeopardize my career and my children's future. I explained this to Rajinder and the children and informed them that I would not be able to go to India in the near future. My inability to attend occasions as important as my daughters' marriages drove a permanent wedge between us.

By 1969, Surinder had obtained a BSc and BEd and worked as a school teacher. Jag and Awtar eventually got bachelor degrees in engineering, Balbir obtained an MA and an MEd; Jyoti got a DDS; and Nickky reached the BA level. There was no doubt that, as students, they had a much better life than I, but I never told them about my student days and how I had lived in appalling conditions always worried about my next meal and finding the next month's tuition fees.

When Surinder got married, Rajinder wrote asking me to send an absurd amount for the marriage, an amount that I simply could not afford. She, as well as the children, always had a hard time believing me when I told them that I had no savings, that I lead a frugal life in order to send them as much as I did. I went to the Civil Service Co-op and borrowed all that I could, which was about $2,800 or the equivalent of Rs13,000. This amount I then set as the limit for each of my daughters' weddings.

My absence from the wedding did not go unnoticed. Relatives, friends, and neighbors who attended the wedding all asked the same question: "Where is the bride's father?" The embarrassing answer, "He was unable to attend," evoked surprise from many. I discovered later that Rajinder and the children had been pestered with highly personal questions from insensitive relatives who lacked judgment. They gave the verdict of "guilty for being absent," which to them was unpardonable, never mind the reasons. I think that my children, who were still at an impressionable age, also agreed with the verdict.

Balbir got married in November 1972, and Jyoti in October 1976. Again, I could not attend their weddings, and because of my absence, they concluded that I had abandoned them despite my repeated attempts to reassure them. In 1970, Jag, Surinder, and her husband, Harbhajan Mahal, immigrated to the U.S. Soon after their arrival, I went to Cincinnati to visit them. I was delighted to meet Harbhajan. He had been Jag's classmate during their engineering studies. The three lived together in a basement apartment and were full of energy and optimism. I bought them clothes and assured them of my help anytime they needed it.

After marrying Iqbal Bajwa in secret in India, Nickky arrived in Cincinnati unannounced and went to live with Surinder. When she called me, I immediately went to see her. She agreed to pursue her studies at the University of Cincinnati. By 1977, Balbir and her husband, Baldev Dabhia, and Jyoti with her husband, Sarup Gill, had also emigrated and were also living in Cincinnati. Awtar married, and he and his new wife Mina soon followed in their footsteps. (Mina died tragically in a car accident in March 1991. He later married Jasminder, a woman from Punjab.) Jag also married a lovely woman named Kathy. Jag was the leader of the family exodus, which became complete when he sponsored Rajinder and she joined them in Cincinnati.

Rajinder and I had been married 33 years. She had always been hard working, had an excellent temperament, and was always patient and loving with the children. We had been through a lot together and had shared delight in our children. Although our marriage had provided peace and intimacy at times, there had never been passion or sensual gratification. Now, I needed more than what my marriage with Rajinder could offer. My job was permanent, and my future was promising. I was being recognized as a dedicated scientist, had been promoted to levels I had never dared hope to attain.

Before initiating divorce proceedings, I talked to Surinder, Harbhajan, and Jag while on my second visit to Cincinnati. Everybody was dead set against it. Surinder cried the whole time I was there. The reasons were far too difficult for me to explain and remained untold. The divorce became final on December 8, 1971. Rajinder was uncooperative and deeply hurt. Soon after my divorce, I married a woman 18 years younger than I after having known her only for a brief period of time. The union did not last.

Ever since Surinder and Jag first came to the U.S., I visited with my children at least once a year and tried to maintain good relations with them. It was extremely gratifying to see all of them become successful citizens. After Rajinder's death in 1987, Claire accompanied me on these visits. I told my children how much I loved them and tried to convince them that I had done my best to be a responsible father under difficult circumstances that were not entirely of my creation. I tried to explain that obtaining a divorce from their mother had become inevitable. It was a delicate and difficult issue which they found hard to accept. Nevertheless, they listened to me, but offered no response. I could never tell how they truly felt toward me.

I have never compared how I fared as a father with any ideal of fatherhood. Such a comparison would be futile, since I was never able to deal with life on my own terms nor could I avoid all the pitfalls and chaotic circumstances that kept intruding in my life. I do feel badly that I missed out on a major part of my children's lives, and so was denied the opportunity of bonding with them. But, I am extremely proud of all of them and of my grandchildren (I have 16) and see them as a part of myself with strong emotional attachment and a deep sense of family.

During the 24 to 31 years, from the time they arrived in America to the present time, my children seldom visited me in Ottawa or St. Petersburg, Florida, where Claire and I spend our winters. Yet, Claire and I drove almost every year to see them. We enjoyed many family gatherings there since they all live within a 60-mile radius of one another. We also played golf with Jag and Awtar. On every visit, Claire and I were warmly welcomed by all, and everybody rejoiced at the occasion. Every year, I would return home and wonder what happened to all those warm feelings and sincere affection during the rest of the year. I rarely received a phone call, card, or letter enquiring about my health or just to say hello. In sum, our relationship seemed contingent on my visits. From 2001 onward, I stopped going to

Cincinnati, finding that the drive had become too strenuous and tiring. This decision seems to have severed our ties.

My Wife, Claire

I met Claire Paulin on Valentine's Day 1975 at a dance organized by the Single Parents Association. I had skied all day and was in high spirits. I asked her for a dance and was attracted by her happy disposition. As we danced, she sang in tune with the music in a whispering sound as if into my ear. That romantic beginning led to fondness, to deeper feelings of affection and to love. She was 18 years younger than I and had a son, Richard, who was 12, and a daughter, Roxanne, 11, from her first marriage that had ended in a divorce. They all moved into my house in April 1976.

When I met Claire, she was assistant editor with the International Development Research Centre in Ottawa. In 1976, she joined the new North-South Institute as one of the two founding staff members. When she quit working in 1991, she was its Director of Administration and Finance.

Our relationship went through bumpy rides, marked by highs and lows, but we always survived because of the strong bond that we shared and our commitment to each other. In 1986, after being together for ten years, our love and understanding won out, and we were married on March 22 that year. She describes me well in the following poem:

My Husband, the Bookworm
>He sitteth on the balcony
>Day after day
>Reading books of French, history and philosophy;
>He sippeth his tea,
>Dictionary on the lap, markers in hand
>And pens of red, green and blue, and a ruler, too.
>Dare we not interrupt his chain of thought
>With idle chatter or "the box"
>Lest he close the door with a look
>Before he returneth to the book.

For years, I had jogged (up to six miles a day), played tennis, and also dabbled in weight training to increase my strength and tenacity. I also enjoyed skiing, both downhill and cross-country, which made my winters tolerable. But, in 1980, I started having coronary ischemia (angina) which required a quadruple bypass the following year. I had quit smoking in 1966 and rarely drank alcohol. That, plus my fitness level and love of life, helped me sail through the surgery determined to come out a winner. Afterward though, I took up golf because tennis had become too strenuous.

On my coaxing, Claire joined me in playing golf. In the first year, we kept hitting the ball to unintended targets: sand traps, ponds, and bushes around the fairways, always wondering when the fun of this game would start. I soon found out that golf lessons and hitting balls on the golf range were not only expensive, but also highly addictive. Soon, I would be back for more lessons or practice balls after their short therapeutic effects had worn off. For me, golf was always a mystical experience, but for Claire, it was different. She had a natural gift for the game. In her second year, she won her first of many club championships and later twice represented the province of Quebec as a member of the provincial senior ladies team in national championships.

Farming as a Second Job

In the early seventies, I had bought a 165-acre farm in Prescott, about 80 km from Ottawa. It came with a dilapidated farmhouse, a barn in a state of disrepair, and an incomplete new bungalow. Use of the farmland had been abandoned long before, and, as a result, its fence posts had rotted with age and the fences had fallen apart. The fields, overgrown with shrubs and weeds, were surrounded by piles of rocks and boulders probably gathered by early settlers. These stones stood as testimony of the hard manual labor needed to cultivate the land.

The property was isolated, surrounded by about 10,000 acres of brush and woodland owned by the Ontario Government. The whole area with its beautiful trees and gentle hills offered a quiet and peaceful retreat from the bustle of Ottawa. I felt free of pressure and thoroughly enjoyed the sounds of crickets and frogs at night and songbirds at dawn. The glowing fireflies emitting flashes of light were fascinating to watch in the evenings.

Claire, Rick, Roxanne, and I used the whole waste area as recreational land. Claire would pack a lunch, and off we went hiking in the summer, cross-country skiing and snowshoeing in the winter. Every year, we would go out in the fields and cut down our own Christmas tree in preparation for the many memorable Christmas celebrations at the farm with Claire's mother, sisters, brothers, and friends.

Weekends and holidays remained very busy making the farm, which we named "Ganga Cedar Farm" after my mother, a going concern. With money borrowed from the bank, we bought a tractor and other machinery. The barn got a new roof, and its inside was renovated. We also built an addition with four horse stalls with help from Lise, Claire's sister, and her husband Ray.

With the help of a summer student eager to make some money to buy himself a motorcycle, I cut hundreds of fence posts from cedar trees and erected miles of new fences around the property and its interior nine fields. Holes had to be dug in rocky soil, and the fence stretched and stapled to the posts. The fields were cleared of brush with chain saws and a brush cutter and then ploughed and seeded for pasture. Another 30 acres were ploughed, harrowed, and seeded with trefoil and timothy. Harvesting was always very time consuming. Rick, Roxanne, and I and a few summer students or other men sent by Canada Manpower would toil for days, cutting, raking, and hauling the hay into the barn. The year I had open heart surgery, Claire's brother Bob came to do the harvest. It was backbreaking work.

There was no end to the work. The old farm house got a new roof, and the ceiling, walls, and floors were changed. We added a new wood burning stove and converted it into a comfortable home for a caretaker, who would look after the farm during the week.

Then, Claire and I bought two Holstein heifer calves, one for Rick and one for Roxanne. They were named Sunday and Lucky. This was the beginning of our livestock acquisitions. Later, we bought registered polled Herefords, Suffolk sheep, and scrub goats for breeding. We even tried raising pigs, turkeys, and chickens. At one time, we owned 42 cattle, 22 sheep, and 24 goats. This was in addition to Spirit, a lovely red dun purebred quarterhorse mare which I had given to Claire on her birthday. Spirit later gave birth to two fillies, a red dun and a palomino. Rick was a great help on the farm, especially when it came to wrestling down calves or sheep for ear tagging, tattooing, or injecting vitamins and antibiotics.

We enjoyed free-range chickens, ate homegrown lamb and beef, grew vegetables, pickled cucumbers, made pies and soup from pumpkin, converted goat milk into cottage cheese, churned our butter, made yogurt, and had our own apple tree. Farming for us was a vibrant weekend dedication, more for fun than love of labor. From an economic point of view, it was not very profitable. After my open heart surgery in 1981, we decided to sell the animals. So, while I was attending a meeting in Boca Raton, Claire sold the whole lot in one swoop. She met me with the news, a little apprehensive but relieved when she saw how happy I was that they were gone. Regrettably, we also ended up selling the farm in 1989 because we could no longer do all the work needed to maintain the farmland and the outbuildings. We had the farm for almost 17 years – an era rich in memories and nostalgia that live on in our minds.

My Last Word

My life as a scientist was a marathon of solitude and self-discipline. It was far from glamorous, since my name did not travel beyond the memberships of the Toxicology and Teratology Societies. My life was full of hard work and personal sacrifice. Until my retirement, I was so busy that I rarely felt the need for social interactions. Then in 1993, I had to have a triple bypass. This time there were complications, but after a long struggle, I got my health back.

My close call brought back a rush of memories. My brother, Surat, came to spend some time with me during my convalescence. We reminisced. It all came back to me – the community I was born in, its members linked by strong social, religious, and blood ties. Everyone knew each other and cherished their family history. All of us, Muslims, Hindus, and Sikhs, lived and worked together in harmony and celebrated religious functions in peace and goodwill. Strong feelings of togetherness and warm interpersonal relations were the norm in our community. All of us were there to support each other in times of need, casting aside all differences. This strongly influenced my psychological development. When I left India, I left behind my brother Surat, my sister Darshan, Mamoon Jan, cousins, aunts, uncles, and many friends. We are separated by oceans and thousands of miles, but they are always in my memory. I miss their warmth and love.

My emotional ties to Indian culture have remained strong. But I never made a tangible effort to renew or maintain any links with it. I do not celebrate holy days and festivals, although there have been ample opportunities to do so, since Ottawa has vibrant Hindu, Muslim, and Sikh communities, which offer spiritual support, recreation, food, and music. There is a *gurdwara*, a mosque, and a temple which keep our history, culture, and religions alive.

I have struck my roots in Canada to which I owe my undivided allegiance. I have lived here almost half of my life and adapted reasonably well to the North American lifestyle, its music, food, and culture. Since Claire is Catholic, I have often accompanied her in celebrating Christmas and attending other services in her church. I have read up on many religions, and

I respect them all, and better still, I like my own, which has everything that religions have except that there are no revelations, myths, or miracles.

At times, I do feel depressed and embark on a sentimental journey into my past. I listen to Indian music and experience deep nostalgia and a longing for what once was. But always, I reason with myself, look at my life in a positive light, and turn to Claire for support.

My father's abuse made me stubborn and rebellious, but they became positive traits that primed my determination at every rejection and hardened my resolve at every defeat. I got what I always wanted – a steady job and a life of comfort. I never claimed to be a genius and harbored no ambitions of getting rich and famous. I had only a modest dream, that of being happy. I have no internal conflicts. I am happy and at peace with myself.

Genealogical chart

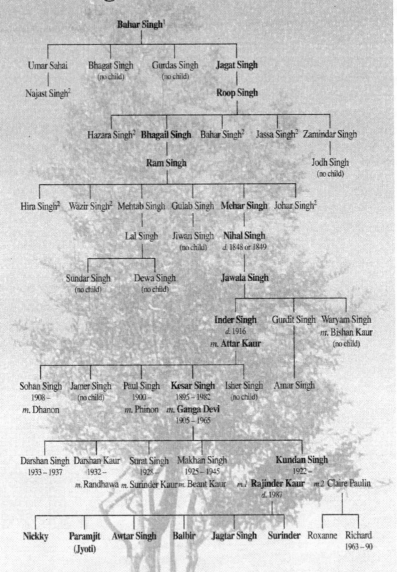

Bahar Singh[1]

- Umar Sahai
  - Najast Singh[2]
- Bhagat Singh (no child)
- Gurdas Singh (no child)
- **Jagat Singh**
  - **Roop Singh**
    - Hazara Singh[2]
    - **Bhagail Singh**
      - **Ram Singh**
        - Hira Singh[2]
        - Wazir Singh[2]
        - Mehtab Singh
          - Lal Singh
            - Sundar Singh (no child)
            - Dewa Singh (no child)
        - Gulab Singh
        - **Mehar Singh**
          - Jiwan Singh (no child)
          - **Nihal Singh** *d.* 1848 or 1849
            - **Jawala Singh**
              - **Inder Singh** *d.* 1916 *m.* **Attar Kaur**
              - Gurdit Singh
              - Waryam Singh *m.* Bishan Kaur (no child)
        - Johar Singh[2]
    - Bahar Singh[2]
    - Jassa Singh[2]
    - Zamindar Singh
      - Jodh Singh (no child)

- Sohan Singh 1908– *m.* Dhanon
- Jamer Singh (no child)
- Paul Singh 1900– *m.* Phinon
- **Kesar Singh** 1895–1982 *m.* **Ganga Devi** 1905–1965
- Isher Singh (no child)
- Amar Singh

- Darshan Singh 1933–1937
- Darshan Kaur 1932– *m.* Randhawa
- Surat Singh 1928– *m.* Surinder Kaur
- Makhan Singh 1925–1945 *m.* Beant Kaur
- **Kundan Singh** 1922– *m.1* **Rajinder Kaur** *d.* 1987 *m.2* Claire Paulin

- Nickky
- **Paramjit** (Jyoti)
- **Awtar Singh**
- **Balbir**
- **Jagtar Singh**
- Surinder
- Roxanne
- Richard 1963–90

[1] Names of male descendents only were available.
[2] Information available but not reported.

198

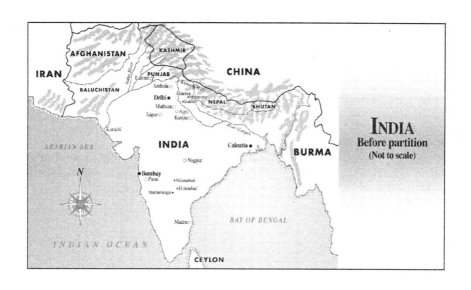

INDIA
Before partition
(Not to scale)

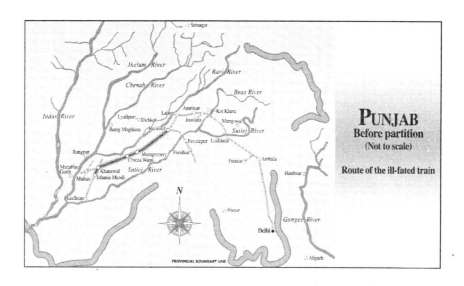

PUNJAB
Before partition
(Not to scale)

Route of the ill-fated train

PROVINCIAL BOUNDARY LINE

Photographs

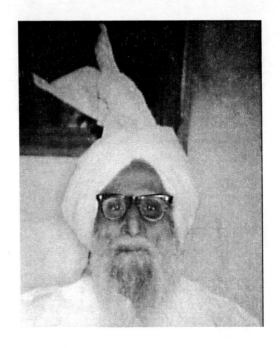

My father, Kesar Singh (1895-1982).

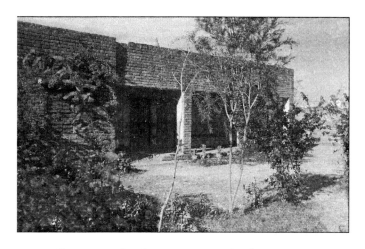

Primary school in Kot Khera built in 1930.

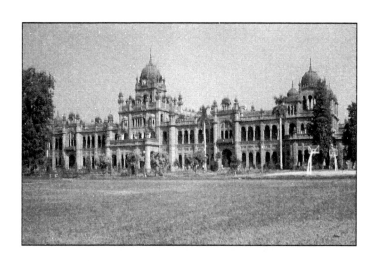

*Khalsa College, Amristar, an educational institution
and centre of Sikh culture.*

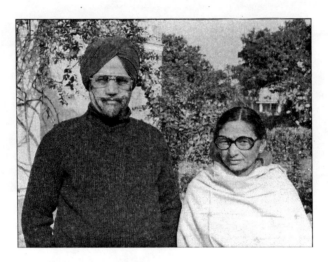

My brother Surat and his wife Surinder.

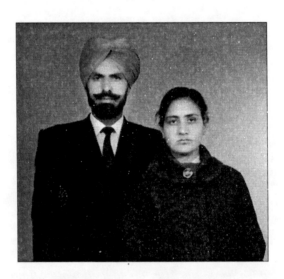

My sister Darshan and her husband Harpal Randhawa.

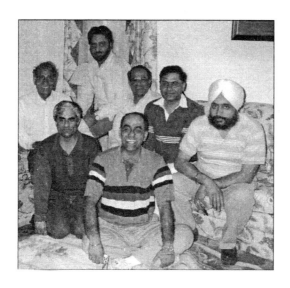

My sons and sons-in-law (left to right, back row): myself, Baldev Dabhia, Harry Mahal, Jagtar, and Sarup Gill; (front row): Iqbal Bajwa and Awtar.

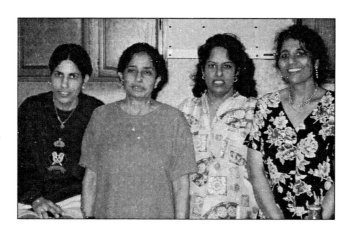

My daughters: (left to right) Jyoti, Surinder, Nickky, and Balbir.

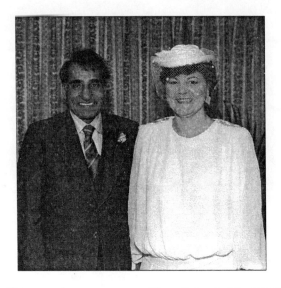

Claire and me at our wedding (March 22, 1986).

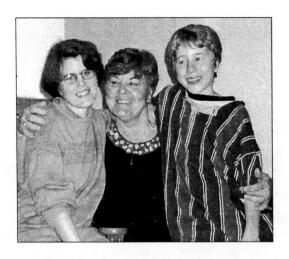

My second family: Claire, Roxanne, and Mich.

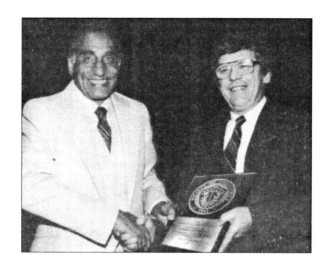

The Arnold J. Lehmann Award presented to me by
Councilor Chris Wilkinson.

Bibliography

Anon. (1970). FDA estimates 23% of canned tuna contaminated by excess mercury, Air/Water Pollut. Rep., *8*:515.

Anon. (1973). Another outbreak of Minamata Disease. Chem. Eng. News, *51*(23):7.

Ban, Y., Nakatsuka, T., and T. Fujii (1989). Correlation between maternal chloride depletion and incidences of fetal wavy ribs in rats. Teratology, *40*:667-8.

Beck, S.L. (1996). Fetal and maternal contributions to differences in valproic acid teratogenicity. Teratology, *53*, 105.

Berriedale, A. Keith (1962). The Age of Rigveda. In: The Cambridge History of India, E.J. Rapson, Ed. S.Chand & Co., New Delhi.

Black, D.L., and T.A. Marks (1992). Role of maternal toxicity in assessing developmental toxicity in animals: A discussion. Regul. Toxicol. Pharmacol., *16*:189-201.

Bligh, E.G. (1970). Mercury and the contamination of fresh water fish, Winnipeg, Fisheries Research Board of Canada Manuscript Report No. 1088.

Branch, C.B. (1970). Testimony presented at the hearing before the sub-committee on commerce, United States Senate, 91st Congress, 2nd session on The Effects of Mercury on Man and Environments, Part 1, Serial 91-73, Washington, D.C., U.S. Government Printing Office.

Bristow, R.C.B. (1974). Memories of the British Raj. A soldier in India. Johnson, London, England.

Burg, David F., and Edward I. Purcell (1998). Almanac of World War I.

Buttar, H.S., Dupuis, I., and K.S. Khera (1978). Dimethadione-induced fetotoxicity in rats. Toxicology, *9*:155-64.

Carson, Rachel (1962). Silent Spring. Houghton Mifflin, Boston, Mass.

Chaudhuri, Nirad C. (1987). Thy Hand, Great Anarchy. London. Chatto & Windus, 19, 283.

Clegg, D.J., and K.S. Khera (1973). The teratogenicity of pesticides, their metabolites and contaminants. Pesticides and the Environment. W.B. Deichmann, Ed., *2*:267-76.

Collins, T.F.X., McLaughlin, J., and G.C. Gray (1972). Teratology study on food colourings. Part I Embryotoxicity of Amaranth (FD&C No. 2) in Rats. Fd. Cosmet. Toxicol., *10*:619-24.

Collins, T.F.X., Welsh, J.J., Black, T.N., and D.I. Ruggles (1983). Teratogenic potential of caffeine ingested in drinking water. Food Chem. Toxicol., *21*:763-77.

Collins, T.F.X., Sprando, R.L., Black, T.N., Shackelford, M.E., Laborde, J.B., Hansen, D.K., Eppley, R.M., Trucksess, M.W., Howard, P.C., Bryant, M.A., Ruggles, D.I., Olejnik, N., and J.I. Rorie (1998). Effects of Fumonisin B_1 in pregnant rats – Part 2. Food Chem. Toxicol., *36*:673-85.

Colomina, M.T., Albina, M.L., Domingo, J.L., and J. Corbella (1995). Effects of maternal stress on methylmercury-induced developmental toxicity in mice. Physiol. Behav., *58*:979-83.

Colomina, M.T., Esparza, J.L., Corbella, J., and J.L. Domingo (1998). The effect of maternal restraint on developmental toxicity of aluminum in mice. Neurotoxicol. Teratol., *20*:651-6.

Copp, T., and W. McAndrew (1990). Battle Exhaustion. Soldiers and Psychiatrists in the Canadian Army. McGill-Queen's University Press.

Cross, Colin (1968). The Fall of the British Empire. Hodder and Stoughton, London.

Cruttwell, C.R.M.F. (1934). A history of the Great War 1914-1918. Academy of Chicago Publishers.

Daston, G.P., Overmann, G.J., Baines, D., Taubeneck, M.W., Lehmanmckeeman, L.D., Rogers, J.M., and C.L. Keen (1994). Altered Zn status by alpha-hederin in the pregnant rat and its relationship to adverse developmental outcome. Reproduc. Toxicol., *8*:15-24.

Datta, S. (1954). The national Rinderpest eradication plan. Ind. J. Vet. Sci. Anim. Husb., *24*:1-10.

DeSesso, J.M., and G.C. Goeringer (1990). Developmental toxicity of hydroxyl amine: an example of a maternally mediated effect. Toxicol. Indust. Health, *6*:109-21.

Dhanda, M.R. (1955-1960). Ind. J. Vet. Sci. Anim. Husb., (1955) *25*:245-53; (1956) *26*:13-20, 273-84; (1957) *27*:79-84, 127-32; (1958) *28*:117-32, 139-56; (1959) *29*:47-56, 57-61, 62-8; (1960) *30*:90-8, 114-35.
Indian Veterinarian, (1958) *1*:13.
Ind. J. Path. Bact., (1959) *2*:59.
Ind. Vet. J., (1959) *36*:6, 327.

D'Itri, Patricia A., and Frank M. D'Itri (1977). Mercury contamination: A human tragedy. John Wiley & Sons, New York.

Document, Carcinogenesis, Mutagenesis, and Teratogenesis (1973). Government of Canada, Queen's Printer, Ottawa, Ontario.

Doi, R., and J. Ui (1975). The distribution of mercury in fish and its form of occurrence. In P.A. Krenkel, Ed., Heavy Metals in the Aquatic Environment, Oxford, Pergamon.

Duffy, J.Y., Baines, D., Overmann, G.J., Keen, C.L., and G.P. Daston (1997). Repeated administration of a-hederin results in alterations in maternal zinc status and adverse developmental outcome in the rat. Teratology, *56*:327-34.

Earl, F.L., Miller E., and E.J. Van Loon (1972). Teratogenic research in Beagle dogs and miniature swine. In: The laboratory animals in drug testing, A. Spiegel, Ed. Fisher, Stuttgart, 233-47.

Encyclopædia Britannica (1962), *12*:174-6; *23*:762.

Environmental Health Criteria 30 (1984). Principals for evaluating health risks to progeny associated with exposure to chemicals during pregnancy. International Programme on Chemical Safety. WHO. Participant (K. S. Khera) in the preparation of the document as a member of the Steering Committee, Task Group and Editorial Committee, 1-177.

Evans, R. (1935). A brief outline of the campaign in Mesopotamia, 1914-1918. Sifton Praed, London.

Farwell, Byron (1989). Armies of the Raj. From Mutiny to Independence, 1858-1947. W.W. Norton & Co., New York.

Fimreite, N., and L.M. Reynolds (1973). Mercury contamination of fish in northwestern Ontario. J. Wildl. Manage., 37, 62.

Foley, G.L., Schlafer, D.H., Elsasser, T.H., and M. Mitchell (1993). Endotoxemia in pregnant cows: Comparisons of maternal and fetal effects utilizing the chronically catheterized fetus. Theriogeneology, *39*:739-62.

FDA (1975). Need to establish the safety of color additives FD&C Red No. 2. Report of the Comptroller of the United States. Food and Drug Administration. MWD-75-40. October 20, 1975.

Gibbs, Philip (1920). Now it can be told. Garden City, New York, 547-8.

Gilbert, Martin (1970). First World War at Last. Macmillan, New York.

Griffin, Lepel, Sir (1968). Cambridge History of India, Volume V, 1497-1858, H.H. Dodwell, Ed.

Grinker, Roy (1945). The medical and psychiatric and social problems of war neuroses. Cincinnati J. Med., *26*:241-59.

Haig, Wolseley, and Richard Burn (1963). Mogul Period, The Cambridge History of India, Vol. IV. S. Chand and Company, Delhi.

Hallett, D.J., Khera, K.S., Stoltz, D.R., Chu, I., Villeneuve, D.C., and G. Trivett (1978). Photomirex: Synthesis and assessment of acute toxicity, tissue distribution, and mutagenicity. J. Agric. Food Chem., *26*:388-91.

Harada, Y.(1968). Congenital (or fetal) Minamata Disease. In: Minamata Disease. Study Group of Minamata Disease, Kumamoto University, Japan.

Harbison, R.D., Khera, K.S., and P.L. Wright (1977). Reproduction and Teratogenesis. In: Principles and procedures for evaluating the toxicity of household substances. National Academy of Sciences, 99-110.

Hasselrot, T.B. (1968). Report on current field investigations concerning the mercury content in fish, bottom sediments, and water. Rep. Inst. Freshwater Res. Drottningholm, *48*:102.

Holden, Wendy (1998). Shell shock. MacMillan, London, England.

House, Charles (1991). FDA tests wheat in 10 states to determine vomitoxin levels. Feedstuffs, *63*(35):1, 3.

House, Charles (1993). Labs, markets try to gauge extent of vomitoxin problem. Feedstuffs, *65*(35):3.

Irukayama, K. (1968). Minamata Disease as a public nuisance. In: Minamata Disease, Study Group of Minamata Disease, Kumamoto University, Japan.

Iverson, F., Khera, K.S., and S.L. Hierlihy (1980). In vivo and in vitro metabolism of ethylenethiourea in the rat and in the cat. Toxicol. Appl. Pharmacol., *52*:16-21.

Johnels, A.F., Olsson, M., and T. Westermark (1967). Mercury in fish: investigations on mercury levels in Swedish fish. Var. Foeda, *19*:67.

Khera, K.S. (1958). Etude histologique de la peste bovine: I. Pathogenèse du virus de la peste bovine dans les ganglions lymphatiques. II. Lésions histologiques au niveau du tractus digestif. III. Lésions dans les différents organes. Rev. d'Elev. Med. Vet. Pays Trop., *11*:399-420.

Khera, K.S. (1958a). Effet cytopathogène du virus de la Fièvre Aptheuse en couche monocellulaire de rein de porc. Ann. Inst. Pasteur, *95*:385-93.

Khera, K.S., and J. Maurin (1958). Etude par la méthode des plaques du virus aptheux (type c) en couche monocellulaire de rein de porcelet. Ann. Inst. Pasteur, *95*:557-67.

Khera, K.S. (1959). Studies on Foot-and-Mouth disease virus (type 0) by plaque assay technique. Ind. Vet. J., *36*:231-6.

Khera, K.S. (1959a). Hemorrhagic encephalomyelitis in sheep and goats associated with focal encephalomalacia (Lumbar Paralysis): A disease of unknown aetiology. Ind. Vet. J., *36*:519-27.

Khera, K.S. (1962). FOOT-AND-MOUTH disease virus: antibody response of goats after natural outbreak and artificial infection of Foot-and-Mouth disease. Ind. Vet. J., *39*:465-72.

Khera, K.S. (1962a). FOOT-AND-MOUTH disease virus: Effect on the virulence of Foot-and-Mouth disease virus (Type Asia 1) serially passaged in goat kidney monolayers. Ind. Vet. J., *39*:523-7.

Khera, K.S., and S.S. Dhillon (1962). Morphology of goat kidney monolayer cultures and cellular changes produced by Foot-and-Mouth disease virus. Am. J. Vet. Res., *23*:1294-9.

Khera, K.S., and S.S. Dhillon (1963). Growth and identification of field strains of Foot-and-Mouth disease virus in goat kidney cultures. Am. J. Vet. Res., *24*:187-92.

Khera, K.S., Ashkenazi, A., Rapp, F., and J.L. Melnick (1963). Immunity in hamsters to cells transformed in vitro and in vivo by SV40: Tests for antigenic relationship among the Papovaviruses. J. Immunol., *91*:604-13.

Khera, K.S., and Q.N. LaHam (1965). Cholinesterases and motor end-plates in developing duck skeletal muscle. J. Histochem. Cytochem., *13*:559-65.

Khera, K.S., LaHam, Q.N., and H.C. Grice (1965). Toxic effects in ducklings hatched from embryos inoculated with EPN or Systox. Fd. Cosmet. Toxicol., *3*:581-6.

Khera, K.S. (1966). Toxic and teratogenic effects of insecticides in duck and chick embryos. Toxicol. Appl. Pharmacol., *8*:345.

Khera, K.S., LaHam, Q.N., Ellis, C.F.G., Zawidzka, Z.Z., and H.C. Grice (1966). Foot Deformity in ducks from injection of EPN during embryogenesis. Toxicol. Appl. Pharmacol., *8*:540-9.

Khera, K.S., and S. Bedok (1967). Effects of thiol phosphates on notochordal and vertebral morphogenesis in chick and duck embryos. Fd. Cosmet Toxicol., *5*:359-65.

Khera, K.S., and D.A. Lyon (1968). Chick and duck embryos in the evaluation of pesticide toxicity. Toxicol. Appl. Pharmacol., *13*:1-15.

Khera, K.S., and D.J. Clegg (1969). Perinatal toxicity of pesticides. Can. Med. Assoc. J., *100*:167-72.

Khera, K.S. (1970). Pathogenesis of undulating ribs; a congenital malformation. Teratology, *3*:204.

Khera, K.S. , Whitta, L.L., and D.J. Clegg (1970). Embryopathic effects of diquat and paraquat in rats. Pesticide Symposia (Wm. B. Diechman, J.L. Radomsky, and R.A. Penalver, Eds.), Halos and Associates, Inc., Miami, Florida.

Khera, K.S., and D.R. Stoltz (1970). Effects of cyclohexylamine on rat fertility. Experientia, *26*:761-2.

Khera, K.S., Stoltz, D.R., Gunner, S.W., Lyon, D.A., and H.C. Grice (1971). Reproduction study in rats orally treated with cyclohexylamine sulfate. Toxicol. Appl. Pharmacol., *18*:263-8.

Khera, K.S., and E.A. Nera (1971). Maternal exposure to methyl mercury and postnatal cerebellar development in mice. Teratology, *4*:233 (Abstract).

Khera, K.S., and W.P. McKinley (1972). Pre- and postnatal studies on 2,4,5-trichlorophenoxyacetic acid, 2,4-dichlorophenoxyacetic acid, their derivatives in rats. Toxicol. Appl. Pharmacol., *22*:14-28.

Khera, K.S. (1973). Reproductive capability of male rats and mice treated with methyl mercury. Toxicol. Appl. Pharmacol., *24*:167-77.

Khera, K.S. (1973a). Ethylenethiourea: Teratogenic study in rats and rabbits. Teratology, *7*:243-52.

Khera, K.S. (1973b). Teratogenic effects of methylmercury in the cat: Note on the use of this species as a model for teratogenicity studies. Teratology, *8*:293-304.

Khera, K.S., and S.A. Tabacova (1973). Effects of methyl mercuric chloride on the progeny of mice and rats treated before and during gestation. Fd. Cosmet. Toxicol., *11*:245-54.

Khera, K.S., and J.A. Ruddick (1973). Polychlorodibenzo-p-dioxin: Perinatal effects and the dominant lethal test in Wistar rats. Advances in Chemistry Series, Number 120.

Khera, K.S. (1974). Teratogenicity and dominant lethal studies on hexachlorobenzene in rats. Fd. Cosmet. Toxicol., *12*:471-7.

Khera, K.S., Iverson, F., Hierlihy, L., Tanner, R., and G. Trivett (1974). Toxicity of methylmercury in the neonate cat. Teratology, *10*:69-76.

Khera, K.S., Przybylski, W., and W.P. McKinley (1974). Implantation and embryonic survival in rats treated with amaranth during gestation. Fd. Cosmet. Toxicol., *12*:507-10.

Khera, K.S. (1975). Fetal cardiovascular defects induced by thalidomide in the cat. Teratology, *11*:65-72.

Khera, K.S. (1975a). Teratogenicity study in rats given high doses of pyridoxine (Vitamin B6) during organogenesis. Experientia, *31*:469.

Khera, K.S., and D.C. Villeneuve (1975). Teratogenicity studies on halogenated benzenes (pentachloro-, pentachloronitro-, and hexabromo-) in rats. Toxicology, *5*:117-22.

Khera, K.S., Villeneuve, D.C., Terry, G., Panopio, L., Nash, L., and G. Trivett (1976). Mirex: A terogenicity, dominant lethal, and distribution study in rats. Fd. Cosmet. Toxicol., *14*:25-9.

Khera, K.S. (1976). The significance of metabolic patterns in teratogenic testing for food safety evaluation. Clin. Toxicol., *9*:773-90.

Khera, K.S. (1976a). Distribution, metabolism, and perinatal toxicity of pesticides with a reference to food safety evaluation: A review of selected literature. In: Advances in Modern Toxicology: New Concepts in Safety Evaluation, (M.A. Mehlman, R.E. Shapiro, and H. Blumenthal, Eds.), 369-420. Hemisphere Publishing, Washington, D.C.

Khera, K.S. (1976b). Teratogenicity studies with methotrexate, aminopterin, and acetylsalicylic acid in domestic cat. Teratology, *14*:21-8.

Khera, K.S., Roberts, G., Trivett, G., Terry, G., and C. Whalen (1976). A teratogenicity study with amaranth in cats. Toxicol. Appl. Pharmacol., *38*:389-98.

Khera, K.S. (1977). Non-teratogenicity of d- and L-goitrin in the rat. Fd. Cosmet. Toxicol., *14*:61-2.

Khera, K.S., and L. Tryphonas (1977). Ethylenethiourea-induced hydrocephalus: Pre- and postnatal pathogenesis in rats. Toxicol. Appl. Pharmacol., *42*:85-97.

Khera, K.S. (1978). Carcinogenicity of food colors. In Carcinogens in Industry and Environments, J.M. Sontag, Ed., Marcel Dekker.

Khera, K.S., and F. Iverson (1978). Toxicity of ethylenethiourea in pregnant cats. Teratology, *18*:311-3.

Khera, K.S., Whalen, C., and G. Trivett (1978). Teratogenicity Studies on Linuron, malathion and methoxychlor in rats. Toxicol. Appl. Pharmacol., *45*:435-44.

Khera, K.S. (1979). A teratogenicity study on hydroxyurea and diphenylhydantoin in cats. Teratology, *20*:447-52.

Khera, K.S. (1979a). Teratogenic and genetic effects of mercury toxicity. In Biochemistry of Mercury, Volume 3, Jerome 0. Nriagu, Ed., Elsevier Biomedical Press, Amsterdam. Chapter 19, 501-18.

Khera, K.S. (1979b). Evaluation of teratogenic effects of dimethoate (Cygon 4E) in the cat. J. Environ. Path. Toxicol., *2*:1283-8.

Khera, K.S., and I. Munro (1979). A review of the specifications and toxicity of synthetic food colors permitted in Canada. Critical Reviews in Toxicology, *6*:81-133.

Khera, K.S., Whalen, C., Angers, G., and G. Trivett (1979). A teratogenicity study on piperonyl butoxide, biphenyl and phosalone in rats. Toxicol. Appl. Pharmacol., *47*:353-8.

Khera, K.S., and B.G. Shah (1979). Failure of zinc acetate to reduce ethylenethiourea-induced teratogenicity in rats. Toxicol. Appl. Pharmacol., *48*:229-35.

Khera, K.S., Whalen, C., Trivett, G., and G. Angers (1979). Teratogenicity studies on pesticidal formulations of dimethoate, diuron and lindane in rats. Bull. Environ. Contamin. Toxicol., *22*:522-9.

Khera, K.S., Whalen, C., Trivett, G., and G. Angers (1979). Teratologic assessment of maleic hydrazide, daminozide, and formulations of ethoxyquin, thiabendazole and naled in rats. J. Environ. Sci. Health, Part B, *14*(6):563-77.

Khera, K.S., and F. Iverson (1980). Hydrocephalus induced by N-nitrosoethylenethiourea in the progeny of rats treated during gestation. Teratology, *21*:367-70.

Khera, K.S. (1981). Common fetal aberrations and their teratologic significance: A review. Fund. Appl. Toxicol., *1*:13-8.

Khera, K.S., and F. Iverson (1981). Effects of pretreatment with SKF-525A, N-methyl-2-thioimidazole, sodium phenobarbital, or methylcholanthrene on ethylenethiourea-induced teratogenicity in rats. Teratology, *24*:131-7.

Khera, K.S. (1982). Reduction of teratogenic effects of ethylenethiourea in rats by interaction of sodium nitrite in vivo. Fd. Chem. Toxicol., *20*:273-8.

Khera, K.S., Whalen, C., and G. Angers (1982), Teratogenicity study on pyrethrum and rotenone (natural origin) and ronnel in pregnant rats. J. Toxicol. Environ. Health, *10*:111-9.

Khera, K.S., Whalen, C., Angers, G., Vesonder, R.F. and T. Kuiper-Goodman (1982). Embryotoxicity of 4-deoxynivalenol (vomitoxin) in mice. Bull. Environ. Contam. Toxicol., *29*:487-91.

Khera, K.S., Whalen, C., and F. Iverson (1983). Effects of pretreatment with SKF-525A, N-methyl-2-thioimidazole, sodium phenobarbital, or 3-methylcholanthrene on ethylenethiourea-induced teratogenicity in hamsters. J. Environ. Path. Toxicol., *11*:287-300.

Khera, K.S. (1983). Effects on reproduction and prenatal toxicity of miscellaneous pesticides. In: IARC Monographs on the evaluation of the carcinogenic risk of chemicals to humans. Volume 30, IARC, Lyon, France, 1983.

Khera, K. S. (1984). Maternal toxicity – a possible cause of fetal malformations in mice. Teratology, *29*:411-6.

Khera, K.S. (1984a). Adverse effects in humans and animals of prenatal exposure to selected therapeutic drugs and estimation of embryo-fetal sensitivity of animals for human risk assessment: A review. Issues and Reviews in Teratology, *2*:399-507.

Khera, K.S., Whalen, C., Arnold, D., and P. Scott (1984). Vomitoxin (4-deoxynivalenol): Reproduction studies in mice and rats. Toxicol. Appl. Pharmacol., *74*:345-56.

Khera, K.S., and C. Whalen (1984). Ethylenethiourea-induced hindpaw deformities in mice and effects of metabolic modifiers on their occurrence. Toxicol. Environ. Health, *13*:747-56.

Khera, K.S. (1985). Phenytoin and trimethadione: Pharmacokinetics, embryotoxicity, and maternal toxicity. In: Prevention of Physical and Mental Congenital Defects, Part C. Alan R. Liss, New York, 317-22.

Khera, K.S. (1985a). Maternal toxicity: An etiological factor in causing embryofetal deaths and fetal malformations in rodent-rabbit species. Teratology, *31*:129-53.

Khera, K.S., Cole, R.J., Whalen, C., and J.W. Dorner (1985). Embryotoxicity study on cyclopiazonic acid in mice. Bull. Environ. Contamin. Toxicol., *34*:423-6.

Khera, K.S., and L. Tryphonas (1985). Nerve cell degeneration and progeny survival following ethylenethiourea treatment during pregnancy in rats. Neurotoxicology, *6*:97-102.

Khera, K.S. (1986). Is the site of action of maternal hyperthermia in the mother or fetus? Teratology, *33*:377-8.

Khera, K.S., Whalen, C., and G. Angers (1986). A teratology study on vomitoxin (4-deoxynivalenol) in rabbits. Fd Chem. Toxicol., *24*:421-4.

Khera, K.S, (1987). Maternal toxicity of drugs and metabolic disorders – a possible etiological factor in the intrauterine death and congenital malformations: A critique on human data. C.R.C. Reviews Toxicol., *17*:345-75.

Khera, K.S. (1987a). Neuronal degeneration caused by ethylenethiourea in neuronal cell layers in vitro and fetal rat brain in vivo. Teratology, *36*:87-93.

Khera, K.S. (1987b). Maternal toxicity in humans and animals: effects on fetal development and criteria for detection. Terat. Carcin. Mutag., *7*:287-95.

Khera, K.S. (1987c). Ethylenethiourea: a review of teratogenicity and distribution studies and an assessment of reproduction risk. C.R.C. Reviews Toxicology, *18*:129-39.

Khera, K.S., and C. Whalen (1988). Detection of neuroteratogens with an in vitro cytotoxicity assay using primary monolayers cultured from dissociated foetal rat brains. Toxic. In Vitro, *2*:257-73.

Khera, K.S. (1989). Ethylenethiourea-induced hydrocephalus in vivo and in vitro with a note on the use of a constant gaseous atmosphere for rat embryo cultures. Teratology, *39*:277-85.

Khera, K.S., Grice, H.C., and D.J. Clegg, Eds. (1989). Interpretation and Extrapolation of Reproductive Data to Establish Human Safety Standards. Springer-Verlag, New York.

Khera, K.S. (1990). Response to Daston: Ethylenethiourea: in vivo/in vitro comparison of teratogenicity. Teratology, *41*:477-8.

Khera, K.S. (1991). Chemically-induced alterations in maternal homeostasis and histology of conceptus: their etiologic significance in rat fetal anomalies. Teratology, *44*:259-97.

Khera, K.S. (1992). Letter to the Editor. The "maternal arterial space" in the center of rats' placenta may be venous, not arterial. Teratology, *45*:125-9.

Khera, K.S. (1992a). Valproic acid-induced placental and teratogenic effects in rats. Teratology, *45*:603-10.

Khera, K.S. (1992). Extraembryonic tissue changes induced by 2,3,7,8-tetrachlorodibenzo-*p*-dioxin and 2,3,4,7,8-pentachlorodibenzofuran with a note on direction of maternal blood flow in the labyrinth of C57BL/6N mice. Teratology, *45*:611-27.

Khera, K.S. (1993). A morphologic basis for valproic acid's embryotoxic action in rats. Teratogen. Carcinogen. Mutagen., *12*:277-89.

Khera, K.S. (1993a). Letters: Reply to "comments on the direction of blood flow in the central placental vessel in the rat." Teratology, *47*:5-9.

Khera, K.S. (1993b). Mouse placenta: hemodynamics in the main maternal vessel and histopathologic changes induced by 2-methoxyethanol and 2-methoxyacetic acid following maternal dosing. Teratology, *47*:299-310.

Kitamura, S. (1968). Determination on mercury content in bodies of inhabitants, cats, fishes, and shells in Minamata district and in the mud of Minamata Bay. In: Minamata Disease, Study Group on Minamata Disease, Kumamoto University, Japan.

Larsson, K.S., Elwin, C.E., Gabrielsson, J., Paalzow, L.,and C.A. Wachmeister (1982). Do teratogenic tests serve their objectives? Lancet, *2*:439.

Leed, Eric J. (1979). No man's land. Combat and identity in World War I. Cambridge University Press, Cambridge, 181-92.

Lenz, W. (1962). Thalidomide and congenital abnormalities. Lancet, *1*:45.

Maurissen, J.P., Hoberman, A.M., Garman, R.H., and T.R. Hanley (2000). Lack of selective developmental neurotoxicity in rat pups from dams treated by gavage with chlorpyrifos. Toxicol. Sci., *57*:250-63.

Maxwell, Judith (2002). Report of the think-tank Canadian Policy Research Network cited by Kathryn May in Ottawa Citizen, Ottawa, Ontario, September 3, A-1 and A-2.

McBride, W.G. (1961). Thalidomide and congenital abnormalities. Lancet, *2*:1358.

McKay, Paul (2002). Ear Witness to History. Ottawa Citizen, Ottawa, Ontario, August 31, I-1.

McLaughlin, J., Jr., Marliac, J.P., Verrett, M.J., Mutchler, M.K., and O.G. Fitzhugh (1963). The injection of chemicals into the yolk sac of fertile eggs prior to incubation as a toxicity test. Toxicol. Appl. Pharmacol. *5*:760-71.

McLaughlin, J., Jr., Marliac, J.P., Verrett, M.J., Mutchler, M.K., and O.G. Fitzhugh (1964). Toxicity of 14 volatile chemicals as measured by the chick embryo method. Am. Ind. Hyg. Assoc. J., *25*:282-3.

Melnick, J.L., Khera, K.S., and F. Rapp (1964). Papovavirus SV40: Failure to isolate infectious virus from transformed hamster cells synthesizing SV40-induced antigens. Virology, *23*:430-2.

Miller, G.E., Grant, P.M., Kishore, R., Steinkruger, F.J., Rowland, F.S., and V.P. Guinn (1972). Mercury concentrations in museum specimens of tuna and swordfish. Science, *175*:1121.

Mitchell, Maj. T.V. (1931). Official History of the Great War. Medical Services Casualties and Medical Statistics, London, England.

Moberly, F.J. (1924). The campaign in Mesopotamia, 1914-1918, Vol. II. His Majesty's Stationery Office, London, England.

Murakami, U. (1972). Organic mercury problem affecting intrauterine life. In: M.A. Klingberg, A. Abramovici, and J. Chemke, Eds. Advances in Experimental Medicine and Biology, Volume 27, New York, Plenum.

Nadolney, C.H., Chernoff, N., Dixon, R.L., Khera, K.S., Krowke, R., Leonov, B.V., Neubert, D., and S. Tabacova (1990). Potential short term tests to detect chemicals capable of causing reproductive and developmental dysfunction. In: Short Term Toxicity Tests for Non-genotoxic Effects, P. Bourdeau, E. Somers, G.M. Richardson and J.R. Hickman, Eds. John Wiley, Toronto, Ontario, 163-75.

Olney, John W. (1969). Brain lesions and other disturbances in mice treated with monosodium glutamate. Science, *164*:719-21.

Ozawa, M., Nakatsuka, T., Ikeda, H., Fujii, T. and T. Sakaguchi (1990). Metabolic alkalosis induced by furosemide in pregnant rats and its relation to the occurrence of fetal wavy ribs. Teratology, *42*:27A.

Perelmutter, L., and K.S. Khera (1969). Rat mast cells in human reagin detection. Lancet, Vol I for 1969, 1259.

Perelmutter, L., and K.S. Khera (1970). A study on the detection of human reagins with rat peritoneal mast cells. Int. Arch. Allergy, *39*:27-44.

Pitt, J.A. (1997). Chemical- or dietary-induced maternal zinc deficiency and developmental toxicity in the New Zealand white rabbit. Diss. Abstr. Int. Sci., *58*:664B.

Prakash, Shri (1988). Congress and Question of Secular Politics in India. The Indian National Congress and the Political Economy of India, Mike Shepperdson and Colin Simmons, Eds., Brookfield, U.S.A., 195-207.

Rapp, F., Khera, K.S., and J.L. Melnick (1964). Resistance of BHK21 hamster cells to SV40 Papovavirus. Nature, *201*:1349-50.

Riese, Walter (1929). Allgemeine Ärtzliche Zeitschrift f. Psychotherapie und Psychologische Hygiene, *2*:741-52 (Cited by Leed, Eric J. (1979). No man's land. Cambridge University Press, Cambridge.)

218

Robertson, Ian (1989). Blue Guide, Paris and Versailles. Norton, New York, 73.

Romer, T.R. (1983). Questions about vomitoxin remain unanswered. Feedstuffs, *55*:30.

Ruddick, J.A., and K.S. Khera (1975). Pattern of anomalies following single oral doses of ethylenethiourea on days 10-21 of gestation in rats. Teratology, *12*:277-81.

Ruddick, J.A., Williams, D.T., Hierlihy, L., and K.S. Khera (1976). ^{14}C-Ethylenethiourea: Distribution, excretion and metabolism in the pregnant rat. Teratology, *13*:35-40.

Scott, P.M. (1980). Joint Mycotoxin Committee Report. Association of Official Analytical Chemists Convention, Washington, D.C., October 23.

Scott, P.M. (1981). Joint Mycotoxin Committee report. Association of Official Analytical Chemists Convention, Washington, D.C., October 22.

Sharova, L., Sura, P., Smith, B.J., Gogal, R.M., Sharov, A.A., Ward, D.L., and S.D. Hollada (2000). Non-specific stimulation of the maternal immune system. II. Effects on gene expression in the fetus. Teratology, *62*: 420-8.

Shtenberg, A.I., and E.V. Gavrilenko (1970). Effects of Amaranth food dye on reproductive function and progeny development in experiments in Albino rats. Vop. Pitan., *29*:66

Singh, Khushwant (1963). A History of the Sikhs, Vol. I, 1469-1839. Princeton University Press, New Delhi.

Singh, Khushwant (1966). A History of the Sikhs, Vol. II, 1839-1974. Oxford University Press, Oxford.

Staples, R.E. (1976). Predictiveness and limitations of test methods in teratology: Overview. Environ. Health Perspect., *18*:95-6.

Stoltz, D.R., Khera, K.S., Bendall, R., and S.W. Gunner (1970). Cytogenetic studies with cyclamate and related compounds. Science, *167*:1501-2.

Sullivan-Jones, P., Hansen, D.K., Sheehan, D.M., and R.R. Holson (1992). The effect of teratogens on maternal cortico-sterone levels and cleft incidence in A/J mice. J. Craniofac. Genet. Dev. Biol., *12*:183-9.

Takeuchi, T. (1972).The relationship between mercury concentrations in hair and the onset of Minamata Disease. In: R. Hartung and B.D. Dinman, Eds., Environmental Mercury Contamination, Ann Arbor Science.

Teratogenesis, Carcinogenesis, Mutagenesis (1987), *7*:287-95.

Terraine, John (1965). The Great War 1914-1918. Macmillan, New York.

Thom, D.A. (1943). War neuroses. Experiences of 1914-1918. J. Lab. Clin. Med., *28*:498-505.

Toxicology and Applied Pharmacology (1988), *94*:177-8.

Townshend, C.V.F. (1920). My Campaign in Mesopotamia. Thornton Butterworth, London.

Tryphonas, L., and K. Khera (1980). Ethylenethiourea-induced hydrocephalus and other CNS malformations – A review. In: New Perspectives in Experimental Teratology, T.V.N. Persand, ed., MTP Press, Lancaster, England.

Tully, Mark, and Jacob Satish (1985). Amritsar: Mrs. Gandhi's last battle. Jonathan Cape, London, *48*:203-6.

Villeneuve, D.C., Grant, D.L., Khera, K., Clegg, D.J., Baer, H., and W.E.J. Phillips (1971). The fetotoxicity of a polychlorinated biphenyl mixture (Aroclor 1254) in the rabbit and in the rat. Environ. Physiol., *1*:67-71.

Villeneuve, D.C., and K.S. Khera (1976). Placental transfer of halogenated benzenes in rats. Env. Physiol. Biochem., *5*:328-31.

Villeneuve, D.C., Felsky, G., Chu, I., Norstrom, R.J., Khera, K.S., and G. Trivett (1979). Photomirex: A teratogenicity and tissue distribution study in the rabbit. J. Env. Sci. Health, *B14*(2):171-80.

Warkany, Joseph (1971). Congenital malformations. Yearbook Medical Publishers, Chicago, 6-19.

Wise, L.D., Cukierski, M.A., Lankas, G.R., and G.L. Skiles (2000). The predominant role of maternal toxicity in lovastatin-induced developmental toxicity. Teratology, *61*:444.

Wobeser, G., Nielson, N.O., Dunlop, R.H., and F.M. Atton (1970). Mercury concentrations in tissues of fish from Saskatchewan River. J. Fish. Res., Bd. Can., *27*:830.

World Health Organisation (WHO) (1968). Methods for Toxicologic Testing of Food Additives, Technical Report Series, No. 144, Geneva, 1-19.

WHO (1975). Technical Report Series, No. 574, Geneva.

WHO (1984). Environmental Health Criteria 30, Principals for evaluating health risks to progeny associated with exposure to chemicals during pregnancy, International Programme on Chemical Safety, Geneva, 1-177.

Yeats-Brown, F. (1945). Martial India. Eyre and Spottiswoode, London, 31.

Oral Presentations and Invited Seminars

Khera, K.S., LaHam, Q.M., and H.C. Grice (1965). Toxic effects induced by inoculation of ENP and Systox into duck eggs. Fourth Annual Meeting of the Society of Toxicology, March 8-10, Williamsburg, Virginia. Abstract: Toxicol. Appl. Pharmacol., 7:488.

Khera, K.S. (1966). Toxic and teratogenic effects of insecticides in duck and chick embryos. Fifth Annual Meeting of Society of Toxicology, March, Williamsburg, Virginia. Abstract: Toxicol. Appl. Pharmacol., 8:345.

Khera, K.S. (1967). Toxic and teratogenic effects of pesticides in duck and chick embryos. Utah State University, Logan, May 22 (Invited).

Khera, K.S. (1967). Altered morphogenesis of notochord and vertebral column in chick and duck embryos treated with thiol phosphates. Annual Meeting of the Teratology Society, May 24-26, Estes Park, Colorado.

Khera, K.S. (1968). Perinatal toxicity of pesticides. Current Views on Pesticides, Food and Drug Directorate Symposium, June 5-6, Ottawa, Ontario (Invited).

Khera, K.S., and L.L. Whitta (1968). Embryopathic effects of diquat and paraquat. Sixth Inter-American Conference on Toxicology and Occupational Medicine, August 26-28; Miami, Florida. Abstract: Ind. Med. Surg., 37:553.

Khera, K.S. (1968). Drug induced malformations in human and experimental animals. Thirty-first Annual Meeting, Ontario Association of Pathologists, October 24-26, Kingston, Ontario (Invited).

Khera, K.S. (1970). Cyclamates and MSG.Regional Consultants Workshop, February 3-5, Ottawa, Ontario.

Khera, K.S. (1970). Pathogenesis of undulating ribs; A congenital malformation. Tenth Annual Meeting of Teratology Society, May 20-22, Annapolis, Maryland. Abstract: Teratology, 3:204.

Khera, K.S., Huston, B.L., and W.P. McKinley (1971). Pre- and postnatal studies on 2,4,5-T, 2,4-D and their derivatives in Wistar rats. Tenth Annual Meeting of Society of Toxicology, March 8, Washington, D.C. Abstract: Toxicol. Appl. Pharmacol., 19:369.

Khera, K.S. (1971). The effects of methyl mercury on male fertility; A comparative study in rats and mice. Second Annual Meeting of Environmental Mutagen Society, March 22, Washington, D.C.

Khera, K.S., and E.A. Nera (1971). Maternal exposure to methyl mercury and postnatal cerebellar development. Eleventh Annual Meeting of Teratology Society, May 2-5, Williamsburg, Virginia. Abstract: Teratology, *4*:233.

Grant, D.L., Villeneuve, D.C., Khera, K.S., Clegg, D.J., and W.E.J. Phillips (1971). Studies on the embryotoxicity and placental transfer of polychlorinated biphenyl (PCB's). Fourteenth Annual Meeting Canadian Federation of Biological Societies, June 15-18, Toronto.

Khera, K.S., and J.A. Ruddick (1971). Perinatal effects of dibenzodioxins in wistar rats. 162nd Meeting of American Chemical Society, September, Washington, D.C. Abstract: Pest., No. 87 (Invited).

Khera, K.S. (1973). Teratogenicity of ethylenethiourea in rats and rabbits. 12th Annual Meeting of Toxicology Society, March 18-22, New York. Abstract: Toxicol. Appl. Pharmacol., *25*:455.

Khera, K.S. (1973). Congenital aspects of male hermaphroditism. Internal Seminar, Toxicology Division, Health Canada, Ottawa, Ontario, April 27.

Khera, K.S. (1973). Effects of methyl mercury in cats after pre- or postnatal treatment. Thirteenth Annual Meeting of Teratology Society, June 13-16, St. Jovite, Québec. Abstract: Teratology, *7*:A-20.

Khera, K.S. (1973). Hazards of drugs to the human fetus. Ontario Regional Meeting, The Royal College of Physicians and Surgeons of Canada. September 20-22, Ottawa, Ontario (Invited).

Khera, K.S. (1973). Selection of laboratory animals for predicting hazards of reproductive organ teratogenesis. 24th Annual Session, American Association of Laboratory Animal Science, October 1-5, Miami Beach, Florida (Invited).

Khera, K.S. (1973). Research Activities of the Teratology Section, Faculty of Pharmacy and Pharmaceutical Sciences, Edmonton, Alberta, November 21 (Invited).

Khera, K.S. (1973). Teratogenicity of drugs: Drug Problems and the Pharmacist, Alberta Pharmaceutical Association, Edmonton, Alberta, November 21 (Invited).

Khera, K.S. (1974). Hexachlorobenzene: Teratogenicity and dominant lethal studies in rats. Annual Meeting of Society of Toxicology, Washington, D.C., March 10-14. Abstract: Toxicol. Appl. Pharmacol., *29*:109.

Khera, K.S. (1974). Women laboratory staff and teratogens: Meeting of Safety Committee, Drug Research Laboratory, Ottawa, Ontario, May 28.

Khera, K.S. (1974). Fetal cardiovascular defects induced by thalidomide in the cat. Fourth Scientific Meeting, Society of Experimental Biology & Medicine, Champlain Section, Ottawa, Ontario, June 1.

Khera, K.S. (1974). Implantation and embryonic survival in rats treated with amaranth during gestation. Meeting of ad hoc Advisory Committee on FD&C Red No. 2, Food and Drug Administration, Washington, D.C., June 6 (Invited).

Khera, K.S., and H.A. Heggtveit (1974). Fetal cardiovascular defects induced by thalidomide in the cat. Fourteenth Annual Meeting of Teratology Society, July 10-13, Vancouver, B.C. Abstract: Teratology, *9*:A-24.

Ruddick, J.A., Williams, I., and K.S. Khera (1974). A teratologic study of single oral doses of ethylenethiourea (ETU) and ^{14}C-ETU in the rat. Fourteenth Annual Meeting of Teratology Society, July 10-13, Vancouver, B.C. Abstract: Teratology, *9*:A-34.

Khera, K.S. (1974). Evaluation of the safety of 2,4,5-trichlorophenoxyacetic acid and 2,3,7,8-tetrachlorodibenzo-p-dioxin. Royal Commission of Inquiry, Pesticides and Herbicides, Vancouver, B.C., October 21, Ottawa, Ontario (Invited).

Khera, K.S., and D.C. Villeneuve (1975). Teratogenicity studies on halogenated benzenes (pentachloro-, pentachloronitro- and hexabromo) in rats. Annual Meeting, Society of Toxicology, March 10-13, Williamsburg, Virginia. Abstract: Toxicol. Appl. Pharmacol., *33*:125.

Villeneuve, D.C., and K.S. Khera (1975). Placental transfer of halogenated benzenes (pentachloro-, pentachloronitro- and hexabromo) in rats. Annual Meeting Society of Toxicology, March 10-13, Williamsburg, Virginia. Abstract: Toxicol. Appl. Pharmacol., *33*:146.

Khera, K.S. (1975). The significance of teratogenic testing in food safety evaluation. International Symposium on Health Effects of Chemicals in Food, May 12-14, Ottawa, Ontario.

Khera, K.S. (1975). Effects of methotrexate and acetylsalicylic acid on cat fetal development. Fifteenth Annual Meeting of Teratology Society, May 11-14, Pocono Manor, Pennsylvania. Abstract: Teratology, *11*:25A.

Ruddick, J.A., Khera, K.S., Williams, D.T. and H. Newsome (1975). Studies into the teratogenic mechanism of ethylenethiourea (ETU) with ^{14}C-ETU and structural related compounds. Fifteenth Annual Meeting of Teratology Society, May 11-14, Pocono Manor, Pennsylvania. Abstract: Teratology, *11*:31A, 32A.

Khera, K.S. (1975). Environmental factors in arthrogryposis. Meeting of the Technical Committee on Arthrogryposis, June 30-July, Calgary, Alberta. Bal, H.S., and K.S. Khera (1975).

Teratogenic effects of ethylenethiourea (ETU) – a degradation product of ethylenebisdithiocarbamate (EBDC) on the rat fetus and urogenital system. Meeting of American Association of Veterinary Anatomists, July 13. Buttar, H.S., Dupuis, I., and K.S. Khera (1976).

Fetotoxicity of trimethadione and paramethadione in rats. Annual Meeting of the Society of Toxicology, March 14-18, Atlanta, Georgia. Abstract: Toxicol. Appl. Pharmacol., *37*:126.

Khera, K.S. (1976). Use of the cat for teratogenicity studies. Annual Meeting of the Society of Toxicology, March 14-18, Atlanta, Georgia. Abstract: Toxicol. Appl. Pharmacol., *37:*149-150.

Khera, K.S., and L. Tryphonas (1976). Ethylenethiourea-induced hydranencephaly in offspring of rats treated during gestation. Annual Meeting of Teratology Society, June 20-23, Carmel, California. Abstract: Teratology, *13*:27A.

Khera, K.S. (1976). Problems in teratology: Selection of animal species and techniques. Symposium on Regulatory Industrial Interphase, August 22-26, Aspen, Colorado (Invited).

Khera, K.S. (1977). Teratogenicity study on hydroxyurea in the cat. Society of Toxicology, Annual Meeting, March 28-30, Toronto, Ontario. Abstract: Toxicol. Appl. Pharmacol., *41*:137.

Tryphonas, L., and K.S. Khera (1977). Postnatal CNS effects of intrauterine exposure to ethylenethiourea in rats. Society of Toxicology, Annual Meeting, March 28-30, Toronto, Ontario. Abstract: Toxicol. Appl. Pharmacol., *41*:143.

Khera, K.S., Whalen, C., and G. Trivett (1978). Teratogenicity studies on linuron, malathion and methoxychlor in rats. Society of Toxicology, Annual Meeting, March 12-16, San Francisco, California. Abstract: Toxicol. Appl. Pharmacol., *45*:344.

Khera, K.S., and F. Iverson (1978). Toxicity of ethylenethiourea in pregnant cat following oral administration at low dosages. Society of Toxicology, Annual Meeting, March 12-16, San Francisco, California. Abstract: Toxicol. Appl. Pharmacol., *45*:290.

Iverson, F., and K. Khera (1978). Ethylenethiourea metabolism in the cat. Blood decay profile and urinary metabolites. Society of Toxicology, Annual Meeting, March 12-16, San Francisco, California. Abstract: Toxicol. Appl. Pharmacol., *45*:225.

Villeneuve, D.C., Khera, K.S., Trivett, G., Norstrom, R., Felsky, G., and I. Chu (1978). Teratogenicity and placental transfer of photomirex in the rabbit. Society of Toxicology, Annual Meeting, March 12-16, San Francisco, California. Abstract: Toxicol. Appl. Pharmacol., *45*:332.

Khera, K.S. (1978). Teratogenic Evaluation of Chemicals, Principle, Technique and Evaluation. Université de Montréal, Montréal, Québec, February 16.

Khera, K.S. (1978). Transplacental Carcinogenesis. Mini Symposium, Toxicology Section, HPB, Ottawa, Ontario, February 23.

Khera, K.S. (1978). Modern concept of Teratogenicity Testing of Chemicals. Iowa State University, Ames, Iowa, March 21.

Khera, K.S., Whalen, C., Trivett, G., and G. Angers (1979). Assessment of the teratogenic potential of biphenyl, ethoxyquin, piperonyl butoxide, Diuron, thiabendazole, phosalone, and lindane in rats. Society of Toxicology, Annual Meeting, March 12-15, New Orleans, Louisiana. Abstract: Toxicol. Appl. Pharmacol., *48*(1) Part 2:A33.

Khera, K.S. (1979). Teratogenic evaluation of commercial formulation of dimethoate (Cygon 4E) in the cat and rat. Society of Toxicology, Annual Meeting, March 12-15, New Orleans, Louisiana. Abstract: Toxicol. Appl. Pharmacol., *48*(1) Part 2:A34.

Khera, K.S. (1979). Protective effect of sodium nitrite on teratogenicity of ethylenethiourea following simultaneous oral treatment of rats. Nineteenth Annual Meeting of the Teratology Society, Sugar Loaf Village, Cedar, Michigan, June 10-14. Abstract: Teratology, *19*:34A.

Khera, K.S. (1979). Biochemical changes in teratogenesis. Symposium on Perspective of Biochemical Toxicology, XI International Congress of Biochemistry, University of Toronto, Toronto, Ontario, July 14 (Invited).

Khera, K.S. (1979). Teratogenic and transplacentally carcinogenic consequences of intragastric nitroso reactions. Workshop on "Sources and Biological Effects of N-Nitroso Compounds." Ottawa, Ontario, November 22-23 (Invited).

Khera, K.S., and F. Iverson (1980). Potentiative action of SKF-525A and N-methyl-2-thioimidazole on ethylenethiourea-induced teratogenicity in rats. Nineteenth Annual Meeting of Society of Toxicology, Washington, D.C., March.

Khera, K.S., Whalen, C., and F. Iverson (1980). Teratogenicity of ethylenethiourea and its potentiation by SKF-525A. Twentieth Annual Meeting of Teratology Society, Wentworth-by-the-Sea, Portsmouth, June 8-12. Abstract: Teratology, *21*: 49A.

Khera, K.S. (1980). Embryological deviations or teratologic effects? Third International Workshop on Caffeine, Hunt Valley, Baltimore, Maryland, October 26-28 (Invited).

Khera, K.S. (1981). Suitability of experimental studies for predicting hazards to human development: Comparison of human and animal data. Toxicology Forum, Annual Winter meeting, Arlington, Virginia, February 16-18 (Invited).

Khera, K.S., Whalen, C., and G. Angers (1981). Teratogenicity study on pyrethrins and rotenone (of natural origin) and ronnel in pregnant rats. Twenty-first Annual Meeting of Teratology Society, Menlo Park, June 20-24. Abstract: Teratology, *23*:45A, 46A.

Khera, K.S. (1982). Impact of nutritional factors on teratology. Nutrition and Toxicology Tripartite, January 18-20, Ottawa, Ontario.

Khera, K.S., Whalen, C., Angers, G., and T. Kuiper-Goodman (1982). Embryotoxicity of 4-deoxynivalenol in mice. Twenty-second Annual Teratology Society Meeting, French Lick, Indiana, June 6-10. Abstract: Teratology, *25*.

Khera, K.S. (1983). Materno-fetal toxicity – a possible cause of fetal malformations. Twenty-third Annual Teratology Society Meeting. Atlantic City, New Jersey, June 26-30. Abstract: Teratology, *27*:56A.

Khera, K.S., and C. Whalen (1983). Teratogenicity of ethylenetheourea in mice and effects of metabolic modifiers on the teratogenic induction. Twenty-third Annual Teratology Society Meeting, Atlantic City, New Jersey, June 26-30. Abstract: Teratology, *27*:57A.

Khera, K.S. (1984). Nerve cell degeneration preceding hydrocephalus in fetal rats following maternal treatment with ethylenethiourea during pregnancy. Twenty-fourth Annual Teratology Society Meeting, Boca Raton, Florida, June 3-7. Abstract: Teratology, 29:41A.

Khera, K.S. (1984). Special Topic – Maternal Toxicity: An important factor causing fetal malformations in small laboratory animals. Twenty-fourth Annual Teratology Society Meeting, Boca Raton, Florida, June 3-7. Abstract: Teratology, 29:11A.

Khera, K.S. (1984). Predictive value of current tests. European Meeting of the Toxicology Forum, Geneva, Switzerland, September 18-22 (Invited).

Khera, K.S. (1985). Association of maternal toxicity with embryofetal death and congenital malformations in humans. Twenty-fifth Annual Meeting of Teratology Society, Callaway Gardens, Pine Mountain, Georgia, July 7-11. Abstract: Teratology, 31:38A.

Khera, K.S. (1986). A survey of the literature comparing maternal toxicity and adverse fetal effects. "Consensus Workshop on the Evaluation of Maternal and Developmental Toxicity." Sheraton-Potomac, Washington, D.C., May 12-14 (Invited).

Khera, K.S. (1986). Comparable neuronal degeneration caused by ethylenethiourea in neuronal monocell layers in vitro and rat fetal brain in vivo. Twenty-sixth Annual Meeting of Teratology Society, Boston, Massachusetts, July 5-9. Abstract: Teratology, 33:39c.

Khera, K.S. (1986). In vitro screening of neuroteratogens in primary monocell layer of neurons cultured from dissociated fetal brains of mice and rats. Twenty-sixth Annual Meeting of Teratology Society, Boston, Mass., July 5-9. Abstract: Teratology, 33:77c.

Khera, K.S. (1986). Extrapolation of teratologic risks from animal data. 14th Annual Conference of European Teratology Society, September 2-4, Ndr. Strandvej, Denmark (Invited).

Khera, K.S. (1986). Maternal toxicity in humans and animals: effects on fetal development, implications in teratology studies and criteria for detection. Public Health Workers. September 5, Copenhagen, Denmark. Abstract: Teratology, 34:403 (Invited).

Khera, K.S. (1987). Absence of a teratologically significant change in the osmolality of amniotic fluid following oral dosing of pregnant rats with ethylenethiourea. Twenty-seventh Annual Meeting of Teratology Society, Rancho Mirage, California, June 14-18. Abstract: Teratology, *35*:63A, 64A.

Khera, K.S. (1988). Ethylenethiourea-induced hydrocephalus in rat embryos: difference between in vivo and in vitro study. Twenty-eighth Annual Meeting, Teratology Society, Palm Beach, Florida, June 12-15:

Khera, K.S. (1989). Drug-induced physiologic changes in maternal arterial blood relevant to embryonal development in rats. Annual Meeting of the Society of Toxicology, Atlanta, Georgia, February 27-March 3.

Khera, K.S. (1989). Specific target systems in in vivo mammalian teratogenicity. Twenty-second symposia, Society of Toxicology of Canada, Montréal, Québec, November 28-29 (Invited).

Khera, K.S. (1990). Ethylene glycol-induced maternal acidosis and hyperosmolality – a possible cause of fetal malformation in rats. Annual Meeting, Society of Toxicology, Miami Beach, Florida, February 10-16.

Khera, K.S. (1990). Role of decidual lesions in cadmium-induced teratogenesis in rats. 9th Annual Ottawa Reproductive Biology Workshop, Ottawa Civic Hospital, Ottawa, Ontario, May 16.

Khera, K.S. (1990). Decidual necrosis and maternal peritonitis as possible contributory factors in cadmium chloride-induced resorptions and malformations upon ip dosing of rats. Thirtieth Annual Meeting, The Teratology Society, Victoria, B.C., June 8-12, Abstract: Teratology, *41*:570-571.

Khera, K.S. (1991). Chemically-induced alterations in maternal homeostasis and conceptal histology: their etiologic significance in rat fetal anomalies. Thirty-first Annual Meeting, the Teratology Society, Boca Raton, Florida, June 22-27, Abstract: Teratology, *43*:414.

Khera, K.S. (1991). Risk assessment of chemical for teratogenic and reproductive effects. International Program on Chemical Safety. Bureau of Chemical Hazards, Ottawa, Ontario, May 6.